GLENCOE

Human Sexuality

Mc
Graw
Hill
Education

About the Author

Mary Bronson, Ph.D., has taught health education in grades K–12, as well as health education methods classes at the undergraduate and graduate levels. As Health Education Specialist for the Dallas School District, Dr. Bronson developed and implemented a district-wide health education program, *Skills for Living,* which was used as a model by the state education agency. She also helped develop and implement the district's Human Growth, Development, and Sexuality program, which won the National PTA's Excellence in Education Award. Dr. Bronson has assisted school districts throughout the country in developing local health education programs. In 1992 and 1998, she was selected as Teacher of the Year by her peers. In 1996 and again in 2000, she was recognized in *Who's Who Among American Teachers*. She is also the author of Glencoe's *Teen Health* textbook series.

connectED.mcgraw-hill.com

Copyright © 2015 McGraw-Hill Education

Send inquiries to:
McGraw-Hill Education
8787 Orion Place
Columbus, OH 43240

ISBN: 978-0-02-140718-7
MHID: 0-02-140718-5

Printed in the United States of America.

1 2 3 4 5 6 7 8 9 QVS 19 18 17 16 15 14

Table of Contents

Sexuality and You

Photo Credit ©Digital Vision/PunchStock

Activating Prior Knowledge

Using Visuals During adolescence, a person's sense of masculinity or femininity develops and matures. In what ways does this process affect a teen's self-image?

Sexuality and Making Responsible Decisions

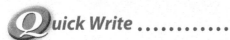**uick Write** ....

People make decisions every day that affect their health. Write a paragraph describing a decision that you recently made concerning your physical, mental/emotional, or social health.

A common theme in books, magazines, movies, and on the Internet, is the use of sexual messages. Advertisers often try to use sexual messages to help them sell their products. These media messages can impact a teen's views on sexual activity. Studies suggest that teens who are exposed to high levels of sexual material in the media are more likely to engage in sexual activity themselves. With that in mind, consider the following:

- Seventy percent of the top 20 TV shows display some form of sexual content.
- On average, a teen will view almost 14,000 sexual references in the media each year.

Even though information on and promotion of sex seem to be everywhere, some people feel uncomfortable talking about sex. To them, sex is a private matter, and they don't talk about it or ask questions about it.

Questions About Sexuality

It's important to have factual information about sexuality issues to help you understand how these issues affect you. This book will address some important issues about sexuality and help you make responsible decisions that protect your health and prevent diseases.

GUIDE TO READING

Building Vocabulary

- sexuality
- self-concept
- goal

Health Concepts

- Identify the physical, mental/emotional, and social changes that occur during adolescence.
- Identify decision-making skills that promote individual, family, and community health.
- Summarize the advantages of seeking advice and feedback when making healthful decisions.

Reading Strategy

Predict Scan the headings, subheadings, and photo captions. Write a list of questions that you have about sexuality.

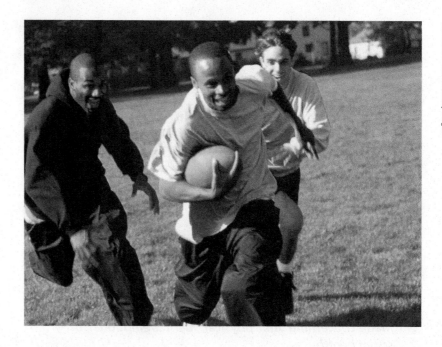

■ **Figure 1.1**
Regular physical activity is one of the keys to good physical health. *What physical activities do you enjoy?*

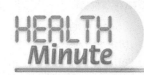

Strategies for Meeting Emotional Needs in Healthy Ways

- Focus on recognizing the things you do well and be willing to improve on areas that can use some attention and effort.

- Pay attention to your feelings and listen to your body.

- Discover interests beyond your school day by getting involved in after-school activities.

- Reach out to help people in need in your community, such as older adults, children, and individuals who need assistance.

Sexuality and Health

Your **sexuality** refers to *everything about you as a male or female. It includes the way you act, your personality, and how you feel about yourself because you are male or female.* Learning about sexuality is an ongoing process that changes as you live, grow, and develop. Your sexuality is an integral part of your health and well-being, including your physical, mental/emotional, and social health.

Physical Health

Good physical health means that you have enough energy to perform the activities of daily life and to cope with every-day stresses and challenges. When you are in good physical health, your body can resist infections and you are more able to protect yourself from injury. Being physically healthy involves:

- Getting at least eight hours of sleep each night.

- Eating nutritious meals.

- Being physically active on a regular basis.

- Drinking up to eight 8-ounce glasses of water each day.

- Avoiding harmful substances, such as tobacco, alcohol, and other drugs.

It is equally important to take care of your reproductive system by practicing healthful behaviors. Practice good hygiene, get regular physical exams, and make responsible decisions that protect against unplanned pregnancy and sexually transmitted diseases.

Mental and Emotional Health

Mental and emotional health relates to how well you adjust and adapt to your surroundings. People with good mental health generally feel good about themselves and tend to be self-confident. They can relate well to other people and are able to cope with life's daily demands. They are tuned in to their feelings and can express themselves in considerate and appropriate ways. They have developed emotional maturity and critical-thinking skills, and are able to use reason.

There is a strong relationship between good mental health and a good **self-concept**, or *the mental image you have about yourself. It is your unique set of perceptions, ideas, and attitudes about yourself.* Beginning in infancy, you receive a variety of signals from people around you that influence how you see yourself. Self-concept is probably the single most important factor influencing what you do. For example, your self-concept influences your ability to make healthy choices. People who respect themselves are more likely to take better care of themselves than people with low self-concepts.

The more protective factors in a person's life, the less likely that person is to seek love and approval by becoming involved in high-risk behaviors, such as engaging in high-risk sexual activity or the use of alcohol, tobacco, and other drugs. Learning to communicate well and to express, understand, and responsibly handle sexual feelings enhances self-concept along with mental and emotional health.

■ **Figure 1.2**
The messages you receive from others help form your self-concept, the mental image you have of yourself. *What other factors help you to live a healthy life?*

Social Health

Adolescence is a time of tremendous change, not only for your body, mind, and emotions, but also for your relationships. During this period, you often begin to examine your values and beliefs and those of your family. You may compare them to those of friends and society at large and start working to shape your own values and standards of behavior into a personal value system that is your own. As you mature, you can benefit from seeking advice and feedback from parents or trusted adults to help you make healthful decisions. This process helps you begin to build your independent identity for the adult world.

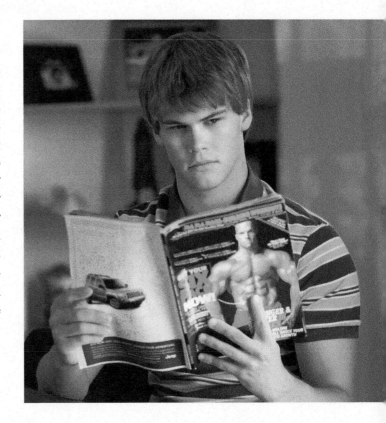

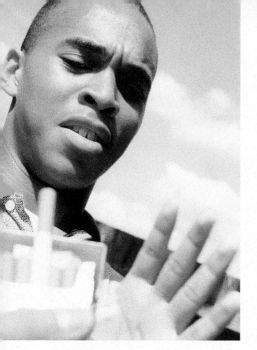

Photo Credit: ©Corbis

■ **Figure 1.3**
When you are faced with a difficult decision, consider your values and ask yourself how you will ultimately feel about that decision.

Making Responsible Decisions

As an adolescent, you are continually faced with choices that can have either positive or negative effects on your overall health. The decisions you make in some of these situations can affect your life for years to come. You need to know how to decide what you should do and consider the consequences to your health and safety.

Decisions, especially about your health and sexuality, can be difficult to make. When you are confronted with a difficult decision, it helps to break the decision down into smaller, more manageable steps. This decision-making model can help you act in ways that promote your health, self-esteem, and respect for others. There are six basic steps in making an important decision.

1. **State the situation.** Be sure the problem is clear in your mind. Ask yourself who is involved, how did the problem develop, and how much time do you have to make a decision?

2. **List the options.** Think of as many ways of solving the problem as you can. Enlist the help of parents, teachers, or trusted friends to get other ideas.

3. **Weigh the possible outcomes.** Consider the consequences of each option, using the word HELP as a guide:
   ▶ **H** (Healthful) What health risks, if any, will this option present?
   ▶ **E** (Ethical) Does this choice reflect what you and your family believe is right?
   ▶ **L** (Legal) Does it violate any local, state, or federal laws?
   ▶ **P** (Parental approval) Would your parents or guardians approve of this choice?

4. **Consider values.** Values are the ideas, beliefs, and attitudes about what is important that help guide the way you live. Consider how each option will reflect your values.

5. **Make a decision and act on it.** Put together all the information you have, make a responsible decision, and act.

6. **Evaluate the decision.** After you have made the decision and taken action, examine the consequences of your decision. How did your decision affect your health and the health of others? Were there any unintended consequences? What did you learn that you would apply in the future?

Goal Setting and Healthy Decisions

A **goal** is *something you aim for that takes planning and work*. Goal setting involves making decisions that will help you meet a goal you have set for yourself. How successfully you meet your goals depends on the decisions you make now. These steps will help you reach your goals.

1. **Select a goal and write it down.** Make it specific, realistic, and something that is important to you and your health.

2. **List the steps you will take to reach your goal.** Break your goal into smaller, short-term goals.

3. **Identify sources of help and support.** Sources might include parents or guardians, other family members, friends, peers, or teachers.

4. **Set a reasonable time frame for reaching your goal.** After deciding on a reasonable time, put it in writing.

5. **Evaluate your progress by establishing checkpoints.** Periodically check your progress and make any necessary adjustments that will help you reach your goal.

6. **Reward yourself after achieving your goal.** Choose a reward that is attainable and healthful.

LESSON 1   ASSESSMENT

After You Read
Reviewing Facts and Vocabulary

1. Define *sexuality* and discuss how it develops.
2. Identify and appraise three areas of health that are affected by changes during adolescence.
3. Define *self-concept* and explain what influences a teen's self-concept.
4. How can you apply the decision-making process to make responsible decisions?

Thinking Critically

5. Synthesize. Make a list of positive mental and emotional changes that occur during adolescence. Describe two specific skills you can develop to promote good physical, mental, and emotional health for yourself, your family, and your community.

6. Analyze. Summarize the advantages of seeking advice and feedback when making healthful decisions. How can a positive self-concept affect decision making? Give two examples.

Applying Health Skills

7. Goal Setting. Think about an important goal related to an extracurricular activity that you would like to achieve. Use the goal-setting process to map out an action plan for working toward your goal. Which decisions were the easiest to make? Which ones were the most difficult?

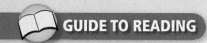

GUIDE TO READING

Building Vocabulary

▸ cognitive
▸ developmental task
▸ empathy

Health Concepts

• Identify the developmental tasks of adolescence.
• Demonstrate strategies for communicating needs, wants, and emotions that lead to responsible behaviors.
• Analyze how changes during adolescence lead to an increased ability to demonstrate empathy toward others.

Reading Strategy

Explain Write the Building Vocabulary terms in your notebook and add a definition written in your own words. After reading the lesson, check your definitions against those in the glossary.

Adolescence and Development

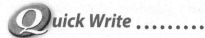

Quick Write

Fold a piece of paper evenly into thirds to make three vertical columns. Label the columns "Physical," "Mental/Emotional," and "Social." Under each heading, write how you have changed since childhood in that category. Write as many specific examples as you can.

During adolescence, physical, mental/emotional, and social changes take place in the human body. As an adolescent, you also experience more subtle cognitive changes that cause you to approach problems in new ways. Everyone goes through this in the process of achieving adulthood. **Cognitive** changes are those *relating to the ability to reason and think out abstract solutions.*

Tasks of Adolescence

Based on the work of Robert Havighurst, a sociologist who specializes in adolescence, there are developmental tasks adolescents must accomplish during their teens and into their twenties. A **developmental task** is *an event that needs to occur during a particular age period for a person to continue his or her growth toward becoming a healthy, mature adult.* These tasks are summarized below:

• Adjusting to and accepting a new physical sense of self
• Adjusting to new intellectual abilities and new cognitive demands at school
• Developing expanded verbal skills to allow for expression of more complex concepts and needs
• Achieving and managing a masculine or feminine social role and a personal sense of identity
• Establishing adult goals of marriage and/or career
• Establishing emotional and psychological independence from parents

- Forming more mature and stable relationships with peers
- Adopting a personal value system and standards of behavior
- Developing a behavioral maturity

Intellectual Development

Until about the age of 12, children think in "concrete" terms, and they believe only what they can see. Consider showing a child two containers that hold exactly the same volume of water but are shaped differently: one container is tall and thin, the other short and wide. If you pour the same amount of water into each container, the child is likely to say that there is more water in the taller container because the water comes up higher in that container. This experiment demonstrates the concrete thinking of the child. As an adolescent, you have bridged that gap between concrete and abstract thought, and now you are capable of more complex thinking:

- **Abstract thinking.** Abstract thinking allows you to analyze and evaluate information, to better understand cause and effect, to examine consequences, and to draw your own conclusions.

- **Logical thinking.** Along with abstract thinking comes growth in mental abilities and an ability to use logic to reason things out. In your head, you can go through the steps from point A to point B and figure out possible consequences.

- **Other, higher-level thinking.** Your ability to see the finer points of an issue increase, and you are also able to remember more. You may find that you are more willing to consider points of view other than your own.

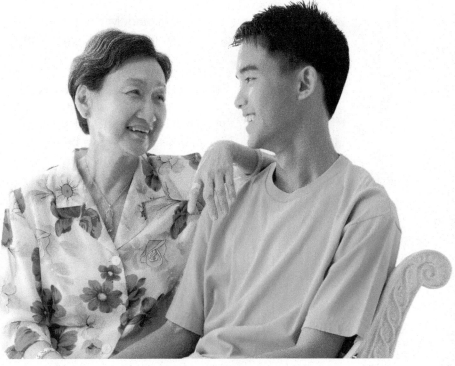

■ **Figure 1.4**
Your ability to think on a higher level increases in adolescence. *How have your verbal skills helped you to show maturity?*

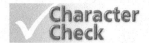
Developing Responsibility

During adolescence, it is natural to work toward achieving independence from your parents or guardians. Teens develop independence in many ways, including the following:

- Taking on a part-time job
- Establishing new goals
- Developing personal values
- Exploring new interests
- Spending more time with friends
- Dating

As this process occurs, you will need to make more decisions on your own and accept the results that come with those decisions. In creating rules and limits, parents teach teens responsibility and consequences. As teens grow closer to adulthood, parents will allow them to make increasingly complex decisions. With each new choice, you become more confident in your decision-making skills. As you make more and more decisions, it is important to remember that you are the one responsible for your choices and that the consequences that follow are your responsibility as well.

Photo Credit: Tim Fuller Photography

Health Skills Activity

Decision Making

Dealing with Peer Pressure

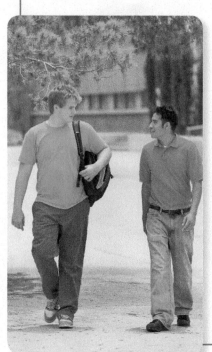

Paul and Mike are walking home after the game on Saturday when Mike's cousin Steve drives up.

"Hey, Mike," Steve calls. "Jump in, guys, we'll give you a ride!" Paul notices that Steve and his friends have beers.

Paul says to his friend, "It's okay, Mike. We are pretty close to home now. I think it's safer if we don't ride with them."

Mike turns to look directly at him. "Aw, come on, Paul, it will be fine."

Paul wonders what he should do.

What Would You Do?

Write a paragraph summarizing how Paul can apply the six steps of the decision-making process to solve his problem.

1. State the situation.
2. List the options.
3. Weigh the possible outcomes.
4. Consider values.
5. Make a decision and act on it.
6. Evaluate the decision.

Developing Mature Relationships

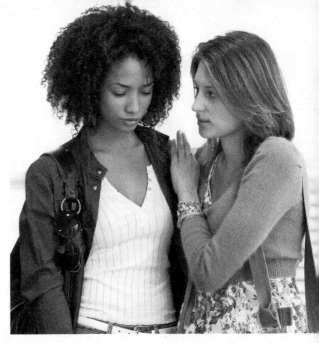

One part of a teen's social development is a growing ability to feel more deeply and consider the needs of other people. This process is crucial to forming more mature peer relationships. As children, most people learn **empathy**, the *ability to feel what others feel, to put yourself in someone else's place.* As an adolescent, you are developing more sensitivity toward others that goes beyond a child's ability to cry when another cries. Your advanced thinking skills allow you to understand the feelings of a friend, and motivate you to want to help your friend resolve whatever it is that is causing distress.

When you demonstrate empathy toward others and offer help, you must always remember to show respect for the other person's feelings, goals, and ideas. Even if you do not share the person's feelings, you can show that you care. Always remember, too, that good friends never urge each other to do something that goes against their beliefs.

Your ability to communicate and express yourself in mature ways will allow you to make responsible decisions in any relationship. When you know how to communicate your feelings, you will be better equipped to avoid unhealthful risk behaviors.

■ **Figure 1.5** Becoming more thoughtful of other people is one of the changes that allows teens to form more mature relationships with their peers.

LESSON 2 ASSESSMENT

After You Read
Reviewing Facts and Vocabulary

1. Define *developmental task*.
2. Name four of the developmental tasks for adolescents suggested by sociologist Robert Havighurst.
3. What process is crucial to forming more mature peer relationships and the ability to demonstrate empathy?

Thinking Critically

4. Evaluate. Review the list of Robert Havighurst's developmental tasks. Which ones do you think would be the most difficult to attain? Explain your reasoning.

5. Analyze. Explain how changes that occur during adolescence lead to increased cognitive abilities and the ability to communicate needs, wants, and emotions. Provide two examples of ways that a teen might show that she is developing more complex thinking abilities.

Applying Health Skills

6. Communication Skills. Write a dialogue in which a teen offers assistance and empathy to a friend who is having a problem. Show how the teen demonstrates empathy and communicates consideration in a respectful way.

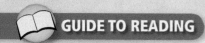
Building Vocabulary

▸ endocrine system
▸ hormones
▸ puberty
▸ pituitary gland

Health Concepts

- Identify the causes of the physical changes that occur during adolescence.
- Explain the role of hormones during puberty.
- Relate the development of secondary sex characteristics to chemical changes that occur within the body.

Reading Strategy

Explain Write a paragraph describing why adolescence is a time of change. What types of physical, mental/emotional, and social changes do adolescents experience?

Adolescence— A Time of Change

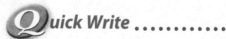

Quick Write

Suppose you have a younger sister or brother age 10 or 11 who is the same gender as you. If your sister or brother asked you what changes they should expect to go through during the next few years, what would you say? Write your answer, and be as specific as possible. Include emotional as well as physical changes.

The body is remarkably complex, with organ systems working together to create and regulate growth, change, flexibility, and stability. The nervous system is the primary regulating system of the body; it works closely with the endocrine system to regulate a variety of body functions.

The **endocrine system** is *a body system made up of ductless glands that secrete chemicals called hormones into the blood.* **Hormones** are *chemical substances produced in glands, which regulate the activities of different body cells and organs.* Hormones control the changes that occur during puberty.

Puberty

During adolescence, hormones signal your body to make the changes that occur during puberty. **Puberty** is *the period of growth from physical childhood to physical adulthood, when a person develops certain traits of his or her own gender.* Puberty is marked by periods of rapid, uneven physical growth, and all teens go through it at their own pace—a pace that is right for each teen's own body. Changes during puberty occur at different times for each individual. The variation in sizes and shapes among people the same age is entirely normal. These changes typically occur between ages 12 and 18. Puberty includes maturing mentally and affects how teens view themselves and others. In addition to body changes, teens also experience emotional changes brought on by the increase in hormones.

Hormones and the Pituitary Gland

Hormones act as chemical stimulators that regulate body functions in three ways:

- **Hormones stimulate reactions in parts of the body.** One reaction is the rush of adrenaline you get in an emergency situation; your heart races, your mouth gets dry, and your palms sweat. You cannot control the secretion of a hormone or your body's reaction to it. Keep this in mind as you learn about other hormonal effects.

- **Hormones produce structural changes in the body during growth periods.** Changes include bone development, maturation of reproductive organs, and development of secondary sex characteristics.

- **Hormones regulate the rate of metabolism.** This is the rate at which body cells produce energy.

The hormones responsible for changes in your body during puberty are released by the pituitary gland. The **pituitary gland** is *the gland that controls much of the endocrine system. It releases hormones that affect the brain, glands, skin, bones, muscles, and reproductive organs.* The pituitary gland is about the size of a pea and is located at the base of the brain. An area of the brain called the hypothalamus stimulates the pituitary gland to release the necessary hormones. The pituitary gland also secretes two hormones that are responsible for stimulating maturation of the reproductive organs that produce sex cells. These organs are the testes in the male and the ovaries in the female. The two hormones are LH (luteinizing hormone) and FSH (follicle-stimulating hormone):

- In the male, LH controls the amount of the hormone testosterone produced by the testes, and FSH controls sperm production.

- In the female, FSH and LH control the levels of the hormones estrogen and progesterone produced by the ovaries; FSH also causes maturation of ova, or eggs, and LH stimulates ovulation—the release of a mature ovum.

■ **Figure 1.6**
During puberty, teens experience growth spurts and other physical changes at different ages and at different rates. *What triggers these changes during adolescence?*

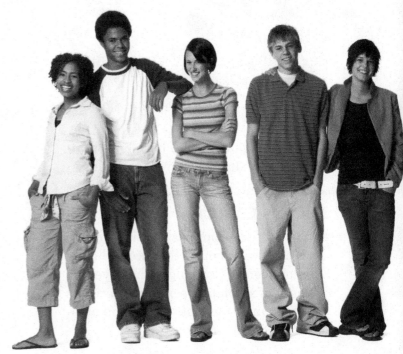

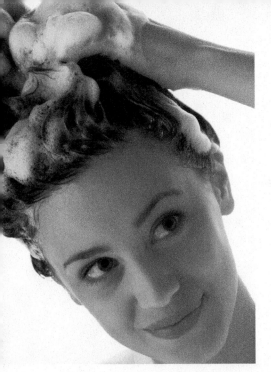

Secondary Sex Characteristics

During puberty, at each teen's own pace, the reproductive organs mature and begin to release the hormones that cause the development of secondary sex characteristics. Secondary sex characteristics are traits that distinguish the two sexes, but are not directly part of the reproductive system. In males, testosterone causes the shoulders to broaden and facial, underarm, and pubic hair to grow. The voice deepens and muscles develop. The bones become longer and larger. In females, estrogen and progesterone cause breast development, growth of underarm and pubic hair, and widened hips.

Along with development of the secondary sex characteristics comes increased activity of the oil and sweat glands. Good hygiene is especially important during this time and will help minimize odor problems.

Concerns over Changes During Puberty

Remember that although adolescents go through all the changes of puberty, each person's time line is different. Growth spurts during puberty depend largely on each person's genetic inheritance and are set in motion by hormones. These hormonal changes cause feelings and sensations never experienced before. It is important to know that everyone grows at a rate that is just right for each individual.

■ **Figure 1.7**
Good hygiene can help to control acne. Medication may be required in severe cases. *Why do you need to pay more attention to personal hygiene during puberty?*

LESSON 3 ASSESSMENT

After You Read
Reviewing Facts and Vocabulary

1. What is the *endocrine system*?
2. What role do hormones play during puberty?
3. Which organs release hormones that cause the development of secondary sex characteristics?

Thinking Critically

4. **Synthesize.** Appraise the significance of physical changes that occur during adolescence. How might the development of secondary sex characteristics affect an adolescent's social and emotional development?

5. **Analyze.** Compare the secondary sex characteristics that develop during puberty for females with those that develop for males.

Applying Health Skills

6. **Stress Management.** A common stressor for teens is to worry over height, weight, or appearance. Make a poster that focuses on how each individual is unique. On the poster, provide a positive tip for handling this stressor, such as thinking positively or being physically active.

Reviewing Facts and Vocabulary

1. Why is it important to have factual information about sexuality?

2. Give one example of a decision that could affect your total health in a positive way.

3. Identify the six steps in the decision-making process.

4. List the goal-setting steps.

5. Define *empathy*.

6. What gland controls much of the endocrine system? Where is it located?

7. Identify the male and female reproductive organs that produce sex cells. Which hormones does each organ release?

8. Name three secondary sex characteristics that occur in males and three that occur in females.

Writing Critically

9. Synthesize. Write a specific example of a decision that could affect your physical, mental/emotional, and social well-being.

10. Apply. Select a goal that you worked toward achieving. Write a one-page analysis comparing and contrasting the steps you took in the goal-setting process. Are there any steps in the process that might have helped you attain your goal?

11. Analyze. Choose three of the developmental tasks based on the work of Robert Havighurst. Write an example of an action you can take to succeed at each of them.

12. Analyze. Write a summary identifying a task that you could not perform when you were a child that, because of cognitive development, you can perform now.

13. Evaluate. Write a letter to help a friend who is depressed because he is shorter than all of his peers.

14. Synthesize. You've noticed that your friend has facial hair that he did not have last year. You've also noticed that he develops body odor by the end of the school day. Create a pamphlet showing teens how to recognize the changes that occur during puberty.

Applying Health Skills

15. Advocacy. Create a pamphlet about the importance of making decisions promoting individual, family, and community health. Include examples of appropriate and effective decision-making skills.

16. Practicing Healthful Behaviors. Write a short story that teaches teens the importance of showing responsibility in caring for their physical, mental/emotional, and social health during adolescence.

Activity Beyond the Classroom

Parent Involvement

Community programs. With the help of your parent or guardian, contact local programs that provide opportunities for teens to volunteer in the community. Create a reference file listing ways that teens can reach out to others while developing their own emotional and social maturity.

School and Community

Endocrine system. Using the Internet or library resources, find out more about the endocrine system. Choose two endocrine glands not discussed in this chapter. Write a paragraph about each gland, describing the hormone each gland produces and the effect of the hormone on the body.

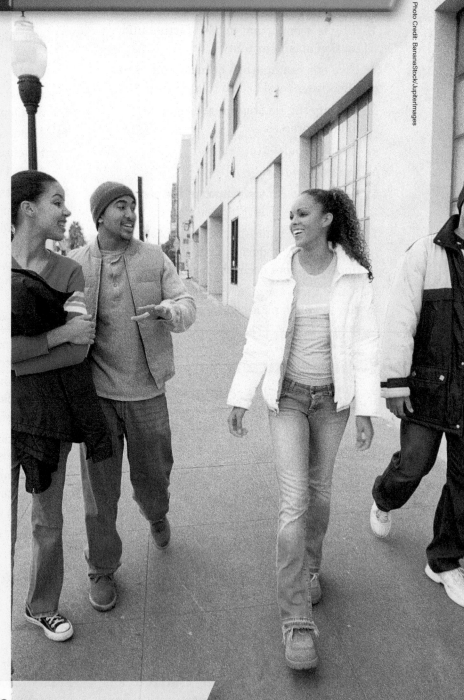

CHAPTER 2

Relationships and Choosing Abstinence

Lesson 1
Relationships and Communication

Lesson 2
Decisions About Sexual Relationships

Photo Credit: BananaStock/JupiterImages

Activating Prior Knowledge

Using Visuals Group dating can help teens feel more relaxed and comfortable in dating situations. What are some additional benefits of group dating?

16

Relationships and Communication

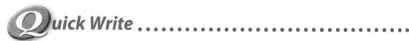

Quick Write ....

List three qualities of healthy relationships. Write one paragraph explaining why those qualities are important and how having healthy relationships can contribute to a fulfilling life.

Humans are social beings. We need other people in our lives. In order to fulfill the basic emotional need to belong, we need to feel that we are valued members of a group. Throughout our lives, we will belong to many different groups.

Family and Friends

The first group that most people belong to is their family. The family is the basic unit of society. Besides ensuring that its members' needs for food, clothing, and shelter are met, the family provides guidance to help children learn to function in society. It is within the family that we first learn to get along with others. Families also teach us our **values**, *the beliefs and standards of conduct that are important to a person.* Values are also instilled through cultural heritage, religious beliefs, and family traditions. You apply your values to the decisions that you make every day.

As we mature, our experience with society increases. We meet people outside of our family, and we begin to make friends and become a part of other groups. These relationships help us learn about ourselves and others. As we get older, our friendships may change. Some friendships may become deeper, while others may change only slightly. Sometimes we may outgrow relationships.

■ Figure 2.1
Friends who share your interests and values can be a source of positive peer pressure. *Describe two ways in which a friend might be a positive influence.*

GUIDE TO READING

Building Vocabulary
▶ values
▶ peer pressure
▶ communication
▶ conflict

Health Concepts
• Evaluate the effects of family relationships on physical, mental/emotional, and social health.
• Evaluate the positive and negative effects of peer relationships.
• Demonstrate communication skills that build and maintain healthy relationships.

Reading Strategy
Organize Create a graphic organizer showing the elements of good communication and good listening skills.

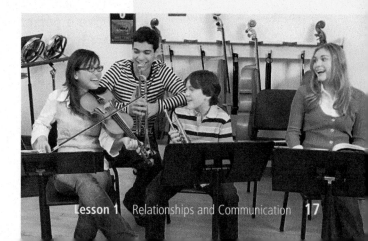

Relationships in Adolescent Years

Many activities during the teen years can broaden and deepen your experience with individuals and groups, helping you to complete this developmental task. Being involved in a variety of school, religious, and community activities can promote your mental/emotional and social growth.

Peer Pressure

As you develop relationships with individuals and groups, you probably will experience peer pressure. **Peer pressure** is *the influence that people your own age may have on you.* Peer pressure can be positive or negative. For example, members of a school club may encourage each other to develop a special talent. However, a person who takes risks may try to persuade a friend to participate in high-risk behaviors such as using drugs or engaging in sexual activity.

Adolescents with low self-esteem can be particularly influenced by peer pressure. In order to feel a sense of belonging, they may engage in high-risk behaviors or other activities that go against their values. Remember that you never have to do anything that makes you uncomfortable. One way to resist negative peer pressure is to surround yourself with friends who share your interests and values. Friends who respect themselves and their well-being are less likely to pressure you into risky behaviors. Also, having friends who promote these positive aspects can influence you to do the same.

Dating

During the teen years, dating is often considered an important social activity. Some teens, however, may not want to begin dating by going on a date with just one person. It's normal to feel uncomfortable and awkward when you first begin dating. Group dates offer teens opportunities to interact with a variety of people while getting to know someone better in an informal setting. Teens may feel less nervous about a first date when they are in a group.

Dating may lead to steady dating, a situation in which two people date each other exclusively. Steady dating may give a person a sense of security, but it may also interfere with developing other healthy relationships. If a relationship doesn't work out, you may think something is wrong with you. This is not true. The other person's interests may change. Although rejection painful, you are worthy of affection.

Declining a Date

At times, you may be asked on a date by someone who you choose not to date. No one should ever feel pressured to date someone you do not want to date. You may feel that you and the other person have different interests or you may have decided that you are not ready to date. Regardless of your reason for saying no, be respectful of that person. Say no, but be kind. If the person persists in asking you on a date, ask him or her to be respectful of your feelings.

Communication

Communication—*the process through which you send messages to and receive messages from others*—is essential to any relationship. Good communication skills will help you keep relationships healthy and form more mature relationships with your peers.

Good Communication Skills

Good communication means clearly expressing your feelings, thoughts, ideas, and expectations. Here are some suggestions for improving your communication skills. Practice these skills when there is no problem in the relationship, and you will be more likely to use them when a problem does arise.

1. Use "I" messages to avoid placing blame.
2. Maintain a polite tone in your voice.
3. Speak directly to the person.
4. Provide a clear, organized message that states the situation.
5. Body language should match your words.

By using "I" messages, you are taking responsibility for how you feel. "You" statements such as, "You are rude when you keep me waiting," send the message that you are blaming someone else.

Did You Know?

Communicating isn't as simple as it seems. Messages can become confusing at any of the following points in an exchange:

- What you intend to say
- What you actually say
- What the other person hears
- What the other person intends to say back
- What the other person actually says back to you
- What you hear

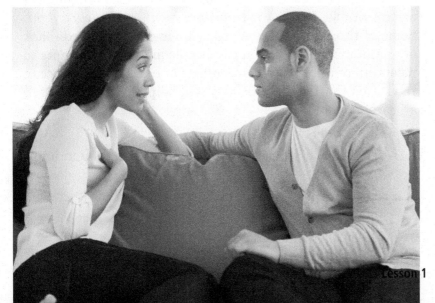

■ **Figure 2.2**
Effective communicators are able to state the situation clearly. *What are other skills effective communicators use?*

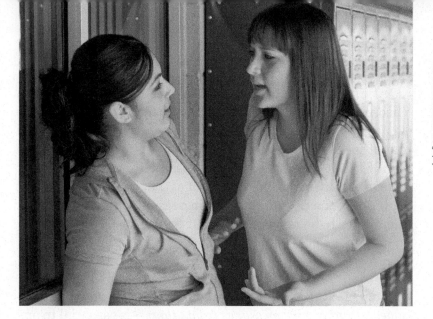

■ **Figure 2.3**
When conflicts occur, remember to stay calm and follow the T.A.L.K. strategy. *Why is it important to take time out if the individuals involved in a conflict are feeling emotional or upset?*

Good Listening Skills

Good communication also means listening to what other people say. Everyone wants to feel that he or she is being heard and is not going to be judged, interrupted, or ignored. Follow these guidelines for being a good listener:

- **Give your full attention to the person speaking.** Eliminate distractions such as a radio or television.
- **Focus on the speaker's message.** Look for the central concept that the speaker is trying to convey.
- **Indicate your interest.** Lean toward the speaker; nod at or encourage the other person. Maintain eye contact.
- **Remember what the speaker has said.** When it's your turn to speak, summarize your understanding of what the other person has said. If you have misunderstood, the speaker can correct you.
- **Use positive body language.** A smile and a nod indicate that you are interested and open to communication.

Conflict

Whether relationships are close or merely casual, conflicts are inevitable. **Conflict** is *a disagreement, struggle, or fight.* Some of the most common reasons for conflict include lack of communication between two people and their attempts to meet different needs. When conflicts or disagreements occur, relying on the T.A.L.K. strategy will help both parties reach a peaceful resolution.

1. **T**—Take time out.
2. **A**—Allow each person to express his or her opinion uninterrupted.
3. **L**—Let each person take turns asking questions and clarifying any statements.
4. **K**—Keep brainstorming to find a good solution.

Compromise, or give-and-take, is essential to every healthy relationship. When both people or both sides feel like winners in a conflict, everyone benefits. For example, friends might agree to alternate activities when spending time together so that each person has a chance to choose an activity.

Conflict and Dating

Becoming skilled at "choosing your battles," or deciding when it is worthwhile to take a stand, can help you avoid unnecessary conflict. Determine if the issue is really important and if it will matter tomorrow, next week, or next month. Thoughtful evaluation of the situation will help you decide if there truly is a conflict. Then you can use the T.A.L.K. strategy to resolve a conflict without compromising your values.

In any relationship, people must communicate in order to have their feelings known and understood. Good communication is especially important in a dating relationship. Both people on a date must be willing to express themselves honestly and listen to what the other person is saying. Suppose you are on a date with someone you really like. Your date wants to see the latest scary movie, but you do not. Do you expect your dating partner to know your preference? How would the other person know? Conflict can occur when two people's expectations are different and are not clearly communicated. Effective communication will help you maintain healthy, mature relationships.

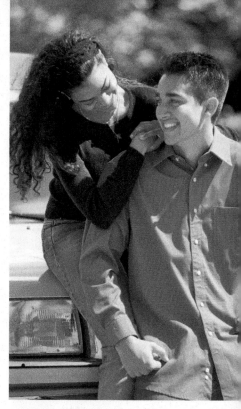

■ **Figure 2.4**
Teens in a dating relationship should identify a variety of activities both can enjoy.
What are other strategies for maintaining a healthy dating relationship?

LESSON 1 ASSESSMENT

After You Read
Reviewing Facts and Vocabulary

1. Evaluate ways your parents, guardians, and other family members contribute to physical and mental/emotional health and help you establish healthy relationships.

2. Define the term *peer pressure* and evaluate the positive and negative effects of relationships with peers.

3. List three benefits of group dating.

Thinking Critically

4. Analyze. Explain and demonstrate the importance of using good communication skills in building and maintaining healthy relationships. Give two examples.

5. Synthesize. Make a list of positive ways you can develop healthy relationships with your peers. Describe specific actions you can take to become a good friend.

Applying Health Skills

6. Analyzing Influences. Divide a sheet of paper into two columns. Label the first column "Family" and the second one "Peers." In each column, list the ways in which that group of people has influenced you in your relationships. Provide at least two specific examples for each column. Evaluate whether the influence on your behavior was positive or negative.

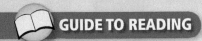
Photo Credit: Tim Fuller Photography

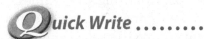
GUIDE TO READING

Building Vocabulary

▶ abstinence
▶ intimacy
▶ refusal skills

Health Concepts

• Analyze the benefits of abstinence from sexual activity.
• Evaluate ways to practice abstinence in a dating relationship.
• Demonstrate refusal skills to reinforce the decision to remain abstinent.

Reading Strategy

Explain Write a summary describing the types of decisions you think teens must make about sexual relationships.

Decisions About Sexual Relationships

*Q*uick Write ....

Describe a decision that a teen in a dating relationship may have to make. Apply the steps of the decision-making process to help the teen make a healthful choice.

When dating, good communication is also critical for setting limits regarding sexual involvement. Each person must decide when he or she is ready to begin a sexual relationship, and communicate those decisions. New and sometimes confusing feelings, especially physical attraction to another person, may complicate how you decide. It is important to recognize that being physically attracted to someone and being in love are not the same thing. Infatuation, or exaggerated feelings of passion for another person, can sometimes be mistaken for love.

Decisions About Sexual Behavior

During your teen years, you will begin making more decisions for yourself. This is part of becoming an adult, but does not mean that you are an adult. One of the choices that you will make is whether to choose **abstinence**, *a deliberate decision to avoid harmful behaviors, including sexual activity and the use of alcohol, tobacco, and other drugs.*

Your family may already have set limits regarding your dating relationships. Remember that seeking advice and feedback from parents or guardians is an important part of the decision-making process as you mature. They can help you determine how to set your own limits.

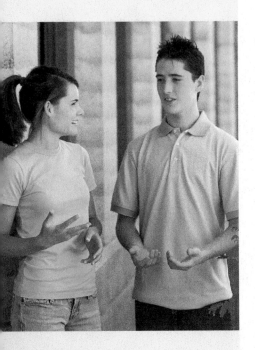

■ **Figure 2.5**
Mature teens effectively communicate their decisions about sexual limits. *What are some healthful ways for dating teens to demonstrate respect for each other's decisions?*

Abstinence from sexual activity is the safe, healthy choice for teens. It is the only method that is 100 percent effective in preventing unplanned pregnancy, sexually transmitted diseases (STDs), and the sexual transmission of HIV/AIDS. However, some abstinent teens may feel pressured by their peers to become sexually active. Sometimes peer pressure may lead teens to boast about imaginary sexual experiences in an attempt to impress others. Keep in mind, that many times these teens are boasting about experiences they have not had. The CDC reports that more than half of U.S. teens are not sexually active.

How can you decide for yourself about remaining abstinent? Ask yourself the following questions:

- Have I communicated with my boyfriend/girlfriend about my expectations in this relationship?
- Do my boyfriend's/girlfriend's beliefs about sexual activity differ from my own?
- Does my boyfriend/girlfriend pressure me to engage in behaviors that I'm uncomfortable with?
- How would I feel about myself if I engaged in sexual activity?
- Am I prepared to deal with an unplanned pregnancy?
- What would I do if I found out I had an STD?
- How would I handle being infected with HIV, the virus that causes AIDS?

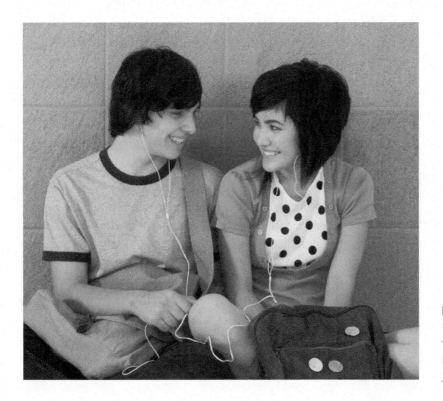

■ **Figure 2.6**
People who choose abstinence take responsibility for their health. *How will abstinence help you reach your goals?*

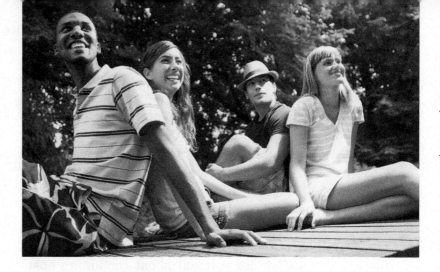

■ Figure 2.7
Practicing abstinence requires genuine commitment. *How can dating in groups help teens keep a commitment to be abstinent?*

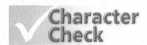

Character Check

Respect **When you make the decision to practice abstinence, you are demonstrating respect for your body.** In what other ways does practicing abstinence demonstrate respect for self and others? Summarize your thoughts in a paragraph.

Practicing Abstinence

By carefully considering and honestly answering the questions on the previous page, many teens make the healthful decision to practice abstinence. Abstinence does not mean there will be no intimacy or physical contact in a relationship. **Intimacy** is *a closeness between two people that develops over time*. For example, a couple can hold hands, hug, kiss, and grow to know and understand each other while practicing abstinence.

Benefits of Abstinence

Young people have identified a variety of reasons to remain abstinent until marriage, including the following benefits to their physical, mental/emotional, and social health:

- Abstinence eliminates both persons' risk of contracting an STD, including HIV/AIDS.
- Abstinence is the only 100 percent effective method to avoid unplanned pregnancy.
- Abstinence ensures that you will not act in a way that goes against your personal values.
- Teens who practice abstinence feel less pressure to continue relationships that are no longer positive or beneficial.

Most teens are not physically, mentally, emotionally, or financially ready for the short-term and long-term consequences of engaging in sexual activity. In addition to the effects on physical and mental/emotional health, there can be legal consequences. It is illegal for an adult to have sexual contact with anyone under the age of consent, which varies from state to state. In many states, it is illegal for unmarried minors to engage in sexual activity.

Practicing Your Decision to Be Abstinent

If you have made the decision to abstain from sexual activity, a well-thought-out plan of action will help you remain committed to that choice. The following steps can help:

- Make a list of your reasons for choosing abstinence.
- Discuss your feelings, your decision, and your expectations of your relationship.
- Place yourself in situations that reinforce your decision to be abstinent. When dating, choose places to go that encourage conversation, or date in groups.
- Plan your time together—where you will go, how long you will stay, and what time you will go home.
- Plan ways to avoid situations that may put your commitment at risk. How will you say no?

Health Skills Activity

Refusal Skills

Communicating a Pledge of Abstinence

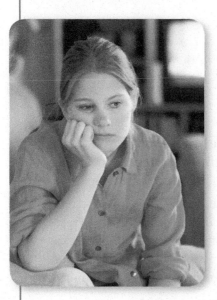

Marla and Dwayne have been dating for several months. Marla is dedicated to remaining abstinent, but she is embarrassed to talk about it with Dwayne. Marla usually tries to plan dates that include activities they both enjoy doing with their friends. Lately, though, Dwayne has been suggesting that they spend more time alone together.

One day, Dwayne tells Marla he loves her. He says that if she really loved him, she would want to add sexual activity to their relationship. Marla cares for Dwayne, but she is also committed to her pledge of abstinence. What can Marla do to communicate effectively to Dwayne her intention to remain abstinent?

What Would You Do?

Use the refusal skills below to write a dialogue between Marla and Dwayne. In the dialogue, Marla remains true to her abstinence pledge and effectively communicates her decision to Dwayne.

1. Say no in a firm voice.
2. Repeat yourself if necessary.
3. Use appropriate body language.
4. If possible, suggest an alternative.
5. Leave if necessary.

Communication in a relationship can be improved if both people understand their rights. In any relationship, you have a right to do the following:

- Make your own decisions.
- Ask for what you want.
- Be treated with respect.
- Say no without feeling guilty.
- Express your thoughts and feelings.
- Protect your health and safety.

Using Refusal Skills

Sometimes, you may feel pressured to make risky decisions that go against your values. In these situations, you will need to firmly say no. Practicing refusal skills will help you uphold your intentions and values. **Refusal skills** are *communication strategies that help you say no effectively when you are urged to take part in behaviors that are unsafe or unhealthful, or go against your values*:

- Say no without feeling that you need to justify yourself. Repeat yourself if necessary.
- Do not insult or yell at the other person, but do use a firm tone of voice and direct eye contact.
- Do not compromise when you feel strongly about something. Compromise can be a passive way of saying yes.
- Avoid the use of alcohol and other drugs. These impair your judgment and your ability to make healthy decisions.
- If the other person persists and continues to pressure you, leave.

Whenever you use refusal skills, congratulate yourself for standing up for what you believe in. You will feel stronger for not compromising your values. Reinforce your decision by reminding yourself that true friends will not challenge you to do something that goes against your values.

LESSON 2 ASSESSMENT

After You Read
Reviewing Facts and Vocabulary

1. Define *abstinence*.
2. Analyze the importance and benefits of abstinence. Discuss how it can promote emotional health and prevent unplanned pregnancy, STDs, and HIV/AIDS.
3. Describe three refusal skills you can use to reinforce a decision to remain abstinent. Give an example of each skill.

Thinking Critically

4. Evaluate. What would you say to a friend who says that he will make a decision about sexual activity when faced with the problem, not before it comes up? Explain your reasoning.
5. Apply. Engaging in sexual activity before marriage can have physical, mental/emotional, and legal consequences. Provide two examples of each of these types of consequences.

Applying Health Skills

6. Practicing Healthful Behaviors. Write a one-act play about someone who is using the refusal skills covered in this lesson to maintain her choice to be abstinent in a dating relationship.

Reviewing Facts and Vocabulary

1. What basic social unit serves as the foundation for your values?
2. Define the term *communication*.
3. Why is it important to use "I" messages when discussing an issue or giving an opinion?
4. List four ways that you can practice good listening skills.
5. Describe the issues that a teen might consider when making decisions about remaining abstinent.
6. What is *intimacy*? Explain how a couple can establish intimacy while practicing abstinence.
7. What aspects of a date can you plan in advance, and how might such planning help you avoid high-risk situations?
8. What are *refusal skills*?

Writing Critically

9. **Synthesize.** Values develop from many different sources, including your family, your religious beliefs, your personal experiences, and your cultural heritage. Make a two-column chart. In the left column, list ten values that are important to you. In the right column, identify the people or experiences that helped you to form these values.
10. **Synthesize.** Write a one-page summary explaining how peer pressure can have a positive or a negative effect on a person's decision to remain abstinent.
11. **Evaluate.** What healthful alternatives would you recommend to someone who is considering giving in to sexual pressure from a girlfriend or boyfriend?
12. **Analyze.** Write a paragraph describing ways that communication skills and refusal skills can help teens maintain healthy dating relationships.
13. **Synthesize.** Jackie has agreed to go to the prom with Ryan. She wants to remain abstinent, but she is extremely attracted to Ryan. She has a feeling that he will pressure her to engage in sexual activity. What advice might you give her?

Applying Health Skills

14. **Communication Skills.** Create a skit with dialogue in which two teens reach an agreement on where to go on a date. Act out the skit with a partner, using polite tones and body language to match the words in the skit.
15. **Decision Making.** Write a short story that teaches teens the importance of making responsible decisions about sexual relationships.
16. **Advocacy.** Create a pamphlet that encourages teens to practice abstinence. Include examples of appropriate and effective communication skills. Be sure to use catchy headlines, graphics, and other visuals to engage the reader.

Activity Beyond the Classroom

Parent Involvement
Group activities. Research where teens in your community can go on group dates that involve safe and healthy activities. Draw a map of your town or city that shows where these places are located.

School and Community
Thinking of the future. Research the difficulties that teens face when they experience an unplanned pregnancy. Find out how having a baby affects a teen's education, finances, and social life.

The Reproductive System

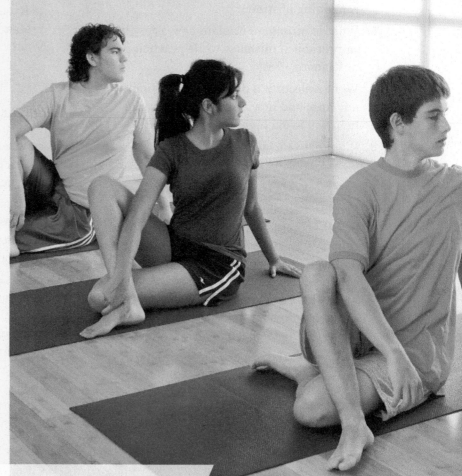

Photo Credit: Tim Fuller Photography

Activating Prior Knowledge

Using Visuals Many changes occur during the teen years. Hormones control these physical and emotional changes. How can keeping your health triangle in balance help you through the changes of adolescence?

The Male Reproductive System

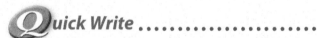

Fold a sheet of paper into thirds. List the external male reproductive organs in the first column. List the internal male reproductive organs in the second column. Write down any questions you have about the structure and function of the male reproductive system in the third column.

The reproductive system produces the cells needed to make a new human being. In this lesson, you will learn how the male reproductive system functions.

External Male Reproductive Organs

The scrotum, the testes (also called testicles), and the penis are the external male reproductive organs. Each has its own role to play in the structure and function of the male reproductive system.

The Scrotum and Testes

Testosterone, *the male sex hormone produced by the testes,* controls the production of **sperm,** *the male reproductive cells.* A mature male can produce millions of sperm daily. To do this, the temperature of the **testes**—*the male sex glands, which produce sperm and manufacture testosterone*—must be a few degrees lower than the normal body temperature of 98.6 degrees F. The **scrotum,** *a loose sac of skin that extends outside the body and contains the testes,* keeps them at the right temperature by holding them either away from or close to the body as needed. When body temperature rises, muscles attached to the scrotum relax, lowering the testes away from the body. When body temperature drops, the muscles tighten and the testes move closer to the body for warmth.

GUIDE TO READING

Building Vocabulary
- testosterone
- sperm
- testes
- scrotum
- epididymis
- penis
- semen
- vas deferens

Health Concepts
- Analyze the relationship between good personal hygiene, health promotion, and disease prevention.
- Describe the function of the male reproductive system.
- Recognize the importance of early detection in the treatment of conditions of the male reproductive system.

Reading Strategy
Organize Information
Create a graphic organizer listing the external and internal male reproductive organs.

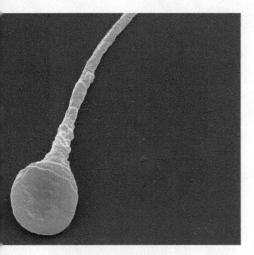

■ Figure 3.1
Sperm can be seen only under a microscope. Each sperm consists of a head, a midpiece, and a tail that moves it through the various ducts and out of the body. *Where are sperm produced?*

Sperm are produced in a section of the testes called the seminiferous tubules. There are about 800 of these thread-like tubes in each testis that produce thousands of sperm every second. Once sperm are produced, they move into the **epididymis**, *a highly coiled structure located on the back side of each testis*. Maturation of the sperm continues in the epididymis and takes about 64 days.

A mature sperm is one of the smallest cells in the body. Each sperm carries 23 chromosomes, half the number present in other body cells. When a sperm unites with a female egg cell, or ovum, which also carries 23 chromosomes, the result is one cell with 46 chromosomes, leading to the production of a human embryo.

The Penis

The **penis** is *a tubelike organ that functions in both sexual reproduction and the elimination of urine*. When sponge-like tissues of the penis fill with blood, the penis becomes enlarged and hard, or erect. Erections are a normal part of being a male, and they occur more easily and more often during puberty.

The penis must be erect for **semen**, *a mixture of sperm and glandular secretions*, to leave the body. The release of semen from the penis is called ejaculation. As many as 300 million to 500 million sperm are released in the average ejaculation. Fertilization—the joining of a male sperm cell and a female egg cell—can result if ejaculation occurs during sexual intercourse. Erection, however, does not mean that semen has to be released; the penis can return to its unerect state without ejaculation.

All male babies are born with a fold of skin, known as foreskin, that covers the end of the penis. Surgical removal of the foreskin is called circumcision. Circumcisions are performed for religious and cultural reasons. For many years, they were also performed because they were thought to be necessary to prevent infection. Doctors now believe circumcision is not medically necessary with good personal hygiene.

Internal Male Reproductive Organs

The internal male reproductive structures play important roles in the male reproductive system. These structures include the vas deferens, the urethra, the seminal vesicles, the prostate gland, and Cowper's glands. These structures are shown in **Figure 3.2** on page 31.

The Vas Deferens and Urethra

After sperm mature in the epididymis of a testis, they travel into the **vas deferens**, *a long tube that connects each epididymis with the urethra*. The urethra exits the body at the tip of the penis. Lined with smooth muscle that contracts to move sperm through the duct, the vas deferens is the main carrier of sperm. Viable sperm can remain in this duct for several months.

The vas deferens loops over the pubic bone, around the bladder, and through the prostate gland. It is 16 to 18 inches long. As it passes through the prostate gland, it narrows and becomes the ejaculatory duct, which opens into the urethra. As sperm travel through these ducts, they mix with several fluids to form semen.

The urethra is a duct that extends 6 to 8 inches from the urinary bladder, through the prostate, and to the tip of the penis. The urethra carries urine from the bladder out of the body; it also carries semen out of the body. Although the urethra carries both urine and semen, it is physically impossible to carry both at the same time. When the penis becomes erect, a ring of muscular tissue closes off the bladder and keeps urine from entering the urethra.

■ **Figure 3.2**
The Male Reproductive System
The male reproductive system includes both external and internal organs.

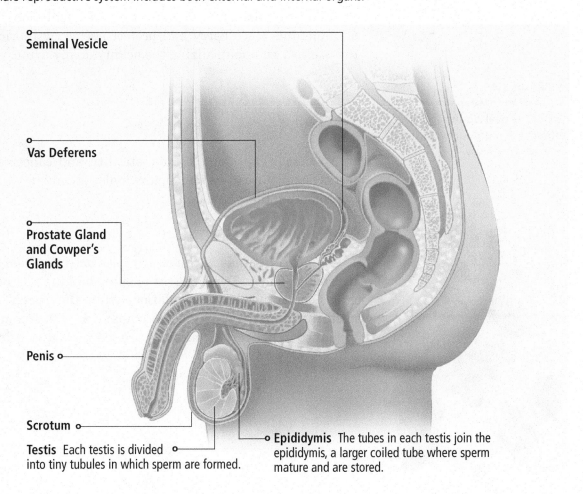

Seminal Vesicle

Vas Deferens

Prostate Gland and Cowper's Glands

Penis

Scrotum

Testis Each testis is divided into tiny tubules in which sperm are formed.

Epididymis The tubes in each testis join the epididymis, a larger coiled tube where sperm mature and are stored.

What is testicular trauma?

Testicular trauma is a painful sensation males experience when the testes are struck, hit, kicked, or crushed, often during sports. Symptoms may include pain, nausea, light-headedness, dizziness, and sweating. If the pain lasts for more than an hour, or if it is accompanied by extreme swelling or discoloration, males should seek medical treatment immediately.

The Reproductive Glands

The purpose of the glands in the reproductive system is to add secretions that support the sperm as they move through the reproductive system. Semen consists of sperm and secretions from the testes, the seminal vesicles, the prostate gland, and Cowper's glands.

The seminal vesicles contribute the most secretions to semen—about 60 percent of the total volume. There are two of these vesicles, or sacs, located on either side of the prostate gland, each measuring about two inches in length. The secretions from the seminal vesicles help make sperm mobile and provide them with nourishment. The secretions from the seminal vesicles empty into the ejaculatory ducts. They then travel into the urethra with the sperm and other testicular secretions, which account for about five percent of the total volume of semen.

The prostate gland lies just below the bladder and surrounds the urethra. It is about the size of a walnut. This gland secretes a milky, alkaline fluid that mixes with sperm. Acids would destroy the sperm, but this fluid helps neutralize the acids found in the urethra and also those encountered in the female's vagina during intercourse. Just below the prostate gland are two pea-sized glands that open into the urethra. Known as Cowper's glands, they secrete a clear mucus into the urethra. This secretion, known as pre-ejaculation, is also alkaline and helps carry and protect sperm by lubricating the urethra and neutralizing the acidity of any urine.

Concerns About the Male Reproductive System

Nocturnal emissions, hernia, sterility, and cancer of the testes or prostate are some factors males should be aware of in promoting their health.

Nocturnal Emissions

In puberty, glands in the male reproductive system begin to produce semen. To relieve the ensuing buildup of pressure, males sometimes have ejaculations while they sleep. These nocturnal emissions may be accompanied by a dream with sexual content. These emissions are also called wet dreams and are perfectly normal.

■ Figure 3.3
Males need to wear proper protective gear during sports to protect the reproductive organs from serious injury.

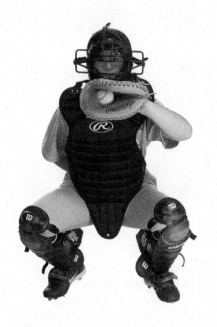

Ken Karp/McGraw-Hill Education

32   Chapter 3   The Reproductive System

Hernia Problems

Males are also prone to hernias, which occur when an internal organ pushes through the wall of muscle that normally holds it in. A common hernia in males is the inguinal hernia. Straining abdominal muscles during activities such as heavy lifting can sometimes cause tears that allow part of the intestine to push through the abdominal wall into the scrotum.

Sterility and STDs

Sterility in a male is the inability to produce offspring. The sperm may be weak, deformed, sparse, or nonexistent. Causes of sterility can include overheating of the testes, exposure to certain chemicals, contracting mumps as an adult, and problems with the epididymis, vas deferens, or urethra. Gonorrhea, syphilis, and genital herpes cause infections that can damage the male reproductive system. Complications of an untreated sexually transmitted disease (STD) can result in male sterility.

Testicular Cancer and Problems of the Prostate

Cancer of the testes occurs most often between the ages of 20 to 34 but can affect a male at any age. The main risk factor for testicular cancer is undescended testes. This condition, where one or both testes remain in the abdomen during fetal development, occurs in about 3 percent of boys. Surgery can correct the problem. The first sign of testicular cancer is usually a lump or the enlargement of a testis. If testicular cancer is found early, the cure rate is very high. Monthly testicular self-examination is important for early detection.

Another type of cancer among men is prostate cancer. After lung cancer, it is the most common cancer in men. Symptoms include frequent or difficult urination, pain when urinating, blood in the urine, or lingering pain in the back, hips, or pelvis. Prostate cancer in boys and young men is rare, and the above symptoms can also be the result of a urinary infection or an STD.

■ **Figure 3.5**
Early detection of testicular
cancer can be accomplished with
a simple three-minute monthly
self-examination.

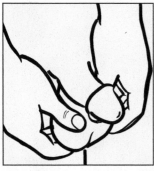

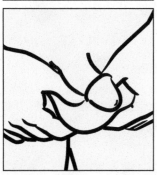

Male Reproductive Health

As the male progresses through puberty and into adulthood, regular medical exams, proper care, and personal hygiene become increasingly important. Regular, thorough washing of the external organs is necessary. Uncircumcised males should pull the fold of the foreskin back and wash under it. A substance called smegma, which is made up of dead cells and glandular secretions, can get trapped under the foreskin and cause irritation or infection.

Other care of the external organs includes a monthly self-examination of the testes. This is best done during or after bathing, when the skin of the scrotum is relaxed. The procedure involves gently rolling each testis between the thumb and fingers. Check for any swelling of the scrotum skin, or lumps on the side of a testis. If there are any hard lumps or nodules on a testis, or if a change in size, shape, or consistency is noted, professional medical attention is necessary. A lump doesn't necessarily mean cancer is present. Only a doctor can determine if a testicular concern is the result of an infection, a possible cancer, or an unrecognized normal structure such as a blood vessel or duct.

LESSON 1 ASSESSMENT

After You Read
Reviewing Facts and Vocabulary

1. Define the terms *scrotum* and *testes* and explain how these parts of the male reproductive system function.

2. List the external and internal male reproductive organs.

3. Analyze the relationship between good personal hygiene, health promotion, and disease prevention. Describe two ways to care for the male reproductive system.

4. Name one disorder of the male reproductive system. Explain why it is important to look for warning signs and seek early detection to prevent disease.

Thinking Critically

5. Synthesize. Describe the route of sperm from the testes to the penis.

6. Evaluate. How might the male reproductive system be affected if the reproductive glands did not function properly?

Applying Health Skills

7. Accessing Information. Using library resources or the Internet, identify one STD and determine how it affects the male reproductive system. Research the symptoms, diagnosis, risks, treatment, and prevention of the disease. Write a paragraph discussing why abstinence from sexual activity is the only 100 percent effective method in the prevention of STDs, including HIV/AIDS. Identify your sources, and explain why you believe they are reliable and accurate.

The Female Reproductive System

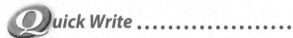

List three facts and three myths you know about the menstrual cycle. Then place a question mark next to each fact that you are unsure about or would like to understand better.

The reproductive system is the only system in the body that has different organs for males and females. The female reproductive system functions to produce mature ova, or egg cells. An egg cell, when united with a sperm cell, forms a fertilized ovum that can develop into a new human being.

External Female Reproductive Organs

Although most of the female reproductive organs are internal, there are some *external female reproductive organs. They consist of the mons pubis, labia majora (outer lips), labia minora (inner lips), vaginal opening, and clitoris.* Collectively, these external organs are known as the **vulva**.

The Mons Pubis and Labia

The mons pubis is a rounded mound of fatty tissue located on the front of the female body, directly over the pubic bone. The labia majora are the fatty outer folds on either side of the vaginal opening. They make up the outer borders of the vulva. Oil and sweat glands on the inner surface of the labia majora provide moisture and lubrication.

Located between the labia majora are two smaller folds of skin known as the labia minora, which contain oil glands and blood vessels. The labia minora also contain many nerve endings and are highly sensitive. The labia serve as a line of protection against pathogens entering the body and also function in sexual arousal. The combined labia majora and labia minora surround the vaginal and urethral openings.

The Vaginal Opening

The vaginal opening lies between the labia minora and may be partially blocked by a thin membrane called the hymen. The hymen usually has several openings in it, allowing for the passage of menstrual flow. The membrane may tear during a variety of physical activities. Hymen tissue is flexible and may stay intact during sexual intercourse. However, sperm released at the vaginal opening can enter the vagina through openings in the hymen, which may result in fertilization and pregnancy. Also between the labia minora, just above the vaginal opening, is the urethra, through which urine is secreted.

Below the mons pubis, where the labia minora meet, is a small knob of tissue called the clitoris. The labia minora form a hoodlike covering over the clitoris. The clitoris plays a major role in female sexual arousal and contains many nerve endings and blood vessels, making it highly sensitive. The clitoris becomes engorged, or filled with blood, during sexual arousal.

Internal Female Reproductive Organs

The internal organs of the female reproductive system are the vagina, uterus, fallopian tubes, and ovaries. The organs of the female reproductive system are shown in **Figure 3.7**.

The Vagina and Uterus

The **vagina** is *an elastic, muscle-lined tube that extends from the uterus to outside the body and is also called the birth canal*. It is three to four inches long and is capable of stretching to allow for the birth of a baby. The vagina is the repository for semen when the male ejaculates with the penis inside the vagina during intercourse. It is possible for sperm to enter the reproductive system if the male ejaculates near the vagina.

The vagina leads to the **cervix**, or *the neck of the uterus*. The cervical opening is quite small. During childbirth, the cervix dilates, or opens up, to allow passage of the baby. The cervix is also the site of glands that secrete mucus to lubricate the vagina. The **uterus** is *a hollow, muscular organ that receives, holds, and nourishes the fertilized ovum during pregnancy*. The uterus is shaped like an upside-down pear and is also about the size of a pear. Its primary function is to hold and nourish a developing embryo and fetus. During pregnancy, the uterus will expand to hold the growing fetus. The uterus has an inner lining called the endometrium, which provides for the attachment of the embryo.

■ **Figure 3.6**
Health care professionals, as well as your parents or guardians, are good sources of information. Medical professionals can answer questions about reproductive health.

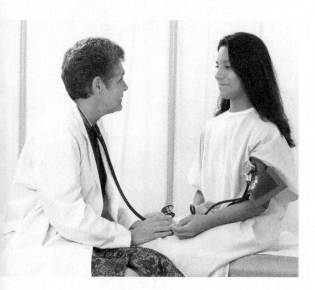

■ **Figure 3.7**

The Female Reproductive System
The female reproductive system provides a place for a fertilized ovum to grow.

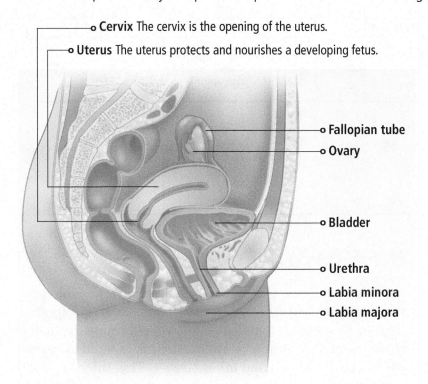

Cervix The cervix is the opening of the uterus.

Uterus The uterus protects and nourishes a developing fetus.

o **Fallopian tube**

o **Ovary**

o **Bladder**

o **Urethra**

o **Labia minora**

o **Labia majora**

The Fallopian Tubes and Ovaries

The **fallopian tubes** are *tubes on each side of the uterus that connect the uterus to the region of the ovaries.* They are extremely narrow and are lined with hairlike projections called cilia. Fingerlike projections at the two ends of the tubes, called fimbriae, surround the top part of the ovaries. The motions of these projections and their cilia gather a released ovum into the fallopian tube. If an ovum is present when sperm enter the fallopian tubes, fertilization may occur. Fertilization of the ovum usually occurs in the widest part of the tube, near the ovaries.

The **ovaries** are *the two female sex glands, which produce mature ova and female hormones.* They are situated on both sides of the uterus, at the open ends of the tubes. In a mature female, the ovaries release ova and produce the hormones that regulate the female reproductive cycle.

At birth, a female usually has hundreds of thousands of immature ova in her ovaries. As she enters puberty, hormones cause the ova to mature; a few hundred will mature during the reproductive years. *The process of releasing one mature ovum each month into a fallopian tube* is called **ovulation.** An ovum can live about a day in the fallopian tube. If sperm are present during this period, and one successfully penetrates the ovum, fertilization has occurred. Pregnancy begins at this point.

The Menstrual Cycle

The menstrual period occurs when an ovum is not fertilized and the lining of the uterus is shed.

Days 1–8	Days 9–13	Day 14	Days 15–28
The cycle begins with the first day of menstruation.	The hormones FSH and LH cause an egg to mature in one of the ovaries.	Ovulation occurs, and the mature egg is released into one of the fallopian tubes.	The egg travels through the fallopian tube to the uterus. If the egg is not fertilized, the cycle begins again.

Illustration Credit: Linda S. Nye

The Menstrual Cycle

With each cycle, the uterus prepares for a possible pregnancy. The typical cycle is 28 days long, but it is important to know that not all females have a regular cycle. Hormones cause the uterine lining, or endometrium, to build up a thick layer of blood vessels and other tissues. This thick layer will support and nourish an embryo if pregnancy occurs. **Figure 3.8** illustrates the typical menstrual cycle.

Menstruation

If pregnancy does not occur, the uterine lining is not needed and begins to break down. The uterus contracts and the lining is shed through the vaginal opening. *The process of shedding the uterine lining* is called **menstruation**. Blood passing out of the body during menstruation amounts to about three to ten tablespoons. This is blood the body does not need; shedding it does not make a person weak or ill. Because the uterus contracts as the lining is shed, the female may experience abdominal cramps during the menstrual period.

The cycle begins when the menstrual period begins. After the menstrual period ends, usually within about five days, hormones signal an ovary to release another ovum around day 14 of the cycle. The uterine lining builds up again, and if pregnancy does not occur, another menstrual period begins.

Most females begin menstruating between the ages of 10 and 15. A healthy female (who is not pregnant) will continue to menstruate fairly regularly until about age 50, when menopause occurs and menstruation ceases.

Did You Know ?

The ovaries make estrogen and progesterone, the hormones that are primarily responsible for the changes females experience during puberty. Before puberty, estrogen and progesterone are secreted in very small amounts.

Menstrual Health Care

Good hygiene is especially important for females during the menstrual period. Daily bathing or showering is very important. If a female uses sanitary pads or panty shields to absorb the menstrual flow, she should change them every few hours. If she uses tampons—cylinders of absorbent material that are placed in the vagina—they must be changed frequently and should not be worn overnight. If she opts to use a menstrual cup, which is a small cup that is put inside the vagina to collect blood, she must empty or replace it every few hours.

Concerns About the Female Reproductive System

Although most females have a healthy reproductive system, it is important for a female to be familiar with her body and know what common problems might occur.

Menstrual Problems

Some females experience premenstrual syndrome (PMS) in the week or two before their period. There are a wide range of symptoms, including anxiety, depression, irritability, bloating, mood swings, and fatigue. PMS symptoms can often be relieved by making healthful changes in one's diet and by increasing physical activity. Severe cases may be treated by a physician or nurse-practitioner with prescribed medications.

Some females suffer from *dysmenorrhea*, or severe menstrual cramps. Menstrual cramps are usually mild to moderate and last only several hours. In some females, the pain may last a day or two. This pain can be controlled with over-the-counter pain medications. Light exercise or a warm bath can be helpful, as can a heating pad placed on the abdomen. In some cases where severe cramping occurs consultation with a medical professional may be necessary.

Amenorrhea is the term for lack of menstruation by age 16 or the stopping of menstruation in a female who previously menstruated and is not pregnant. Amenorrhea can be the result of physical defects in the reproductive organs, diseases such as diabetes, tumors, infections, anorexia, or lack of maturation of the endocrine system. An abnormally low amount of body fat accompanied by excessive exercise, sometimes experienced by professional athletes, can alter hormone levels to a point where ovulation does not occur. A female with amenorrhea should seek professional help to find the cause and correct the problem.

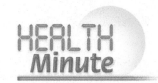

Strategies for Coping with PMS

If you have PMS, your symptoms might include the following:

- Bloating
- Backaches
- Sore breasts
- Depression
- Irritability

These practices can help ease the symptoms of PMS:

- Eating a balanced diet
- Limiting your caffeine intake
- Participating in regular physical activity
- Consulting your doctor or nurse-practitioner if any of these symptoms become severe

Female Infertility and STDs

Female infertility, the inability to become pregnant, has a variety of possible causes. The physical blocking of one or both fallopian tubes, for example, prevents ova from passing into the uterus. In other cases, the female does not ovulate, usually because of a hormonal problem. A third cause of female infertility is endometriosis, a condition in which endometrial (uterine lining) tissue grows outside the uterus in other areas of the pelvic cavity. STDs that are left untreated can also lead to infertility. Untreated gonorrhea and chlamydia are the most common STDs that cause infertility in females.

Problems with Infection

Toxic shock syndrome (TSS) is a rare disease caused by the bacterium *Staphylococcus aureus*. Under certain conditions, the bacterium can produce a toxin that affects the immune system and the liver. Symptoms include sudden onset of fever, chills, vomiting, diarrhea, and a rash. It is believed that using high-absorbency tampons may create an environment in the vagina that allows production of the toxin. Tampons should be changed frequently and used with care. Some contraceptive devices, such as the diaphragm or contraceptive sponge, have also been linked to TSS.

A variety of vaginal infections cause vaginitis, or inflammation of vaginal tissue with discharge, burning, and itching. Yeast infections are caused by a fungus and are generally characterized by a thick, white, odorless discharge accompanied by itching, burning, and painful urination. Yeast infections are rather common and should be diagnosed by a health care professional. Infections may be treated with over-the-counter medications after a definitive diagnosis.

Bacterial vaginosis is the most common type of vaginitis that occurs during the reproductive years. The primary symptom is an odorous vaginal discharge. Trichomoniasis is a vaginal infection caused by a protozoan. Symptoms may include odorous discharge, genital itching, and painful urination. A doctor should be consulted if any of these symptoms occur, so that the organism can be identified and the infection treated.

Cancer

In American females, breast cancer is one of the most common forms of cancer and it is the second leading cause of death, after lung cancer. Two-thirds of cases occur in females older than age 50, but breast cancer can occur in younger females as well. Although it is relatively rare, men also get breast cancer. Early detection through regular medical exams and monthly self-examinations are the best defenses. Chances of surviving breast cancer are much greater when the cancer is found early. Symptoms include a change in breast or nipple appearance, a lump or swelling in the breast, or a lump in the armpit.

Another common cancer in females is cervical cancer. Cervical cancer can be detected by getting a Pap test, which detects abnormal cells. If not caught early, cancer cells can spread to surrounding areas. There are no early symptoms of cervical cancer, but there are several risk factors: being over age 30, not having regular Pap tests, having sexual inter-course at an early age, and having multiple sexual partners. All females should have a Pap test every year beginning at age 18, or earlier if they are sexually active.

Real World CONNECTION

Breast Cancer Statistics

The Internet is an excellent source of information about diseases such as breast cancer, as long as you use reliable sites. How can you tell the site shown below is reliable?

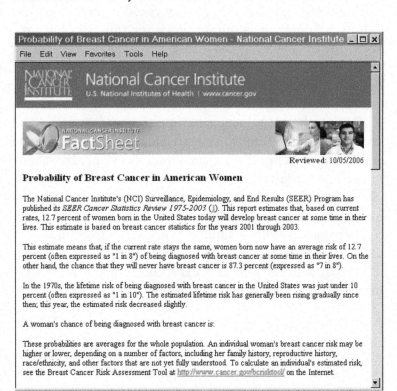

Links to Other Sites

A reputable Web site will provide links so you can learn more about the topic.

Reliable Information

- The most reliable health information is found on sites sponsored by the government, reputable schools and universi-ties, or nonprofit organizations.
- The National Cancer Institute is a government-supported organ-ization that provides the latest scientific research about cancer.
- Commercial sites, such as those maintained by pharmaceutical companies, might have accurate information, but be alert to bias in their reporting.

Reputable Sources

A reputable site will use information from respected journals and from experts in the field.

In the United States, a female's risk of developing breast cancer sometime during her life is calculated to be 1 in 8. For each of the four decades represented, express the risk as a percentage. Graph your results and describe the trend.

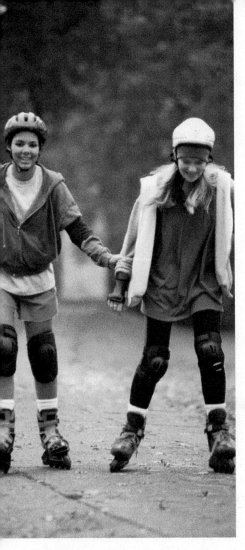

Approximately 20,000 American females are diagnosed with ovarian cancer each year. More than 14,000 die from this cancer annually. The symptoms of ovarian cancer are similar to symptoms for other diseases, making it difficult to detect. They include abdominal pressure, bloating, or discomfort; nausea, indigestion, or gas; frequent urination, constipation, or diarrhea. Ovarian cancer causes abnormal bleeding, unusual fatigue, unexplained weight gain or loss, and shortness of breath.

Photo Credit: Doug Menuez/Getty Images

Female Reproductive Health

In a mature female, the cells in the lining of the vagina are constantly being shed. This often causes a slight vaginal discharge. Bathing regularly, including washing the external female reproductive organs, is an important part of good hygiene. Douches and feminine hygiene sprays are not necessary and may be irritating. Change pads or tampons often. Good personal hygiene and regular professional and self-examinations are important.

Pelvic Examination

The American Cancer Society recommends that females start yearly pelvic examinations after they become sexually active, or by age 21 at the latest. For females up to age 29, a pelvic exam, or Pap test, is recommended every three years. Between ages 30–65 a Pap test is recommended every five years.

During the actual examination, the breasts and abdomen are checked for lumps. The physician checks the external genitalia for general structure and tissue health, then performs an examination of the vagina. To help hold the walls of the vagina apart, an instrument called a speculum is inserted into the vagina. This should be a painless procedure, but because the vaginal muscles are strong, being tense may cause some discomfort. With the speculum in place, the physician collects cells from the cervix for a Pap test. This usually completes the examination.

Breast Self-Examination

Females should perform a breast self-exam (BSE) every month. The best time is right after the menstrual period, when breasts are not tender or swollen. After age 40, an annual mammogram—a series of X-rays of the breasts—is recommended in addition to the BSE. See **Figure 3.10** for how to perform a BSE.

■ **Figure 3.9**
Getting regular physical activity and good nutrition, along with regular medical checkups, are ways to keep the reproductive system healthy.

Early detection of breast cancer can be accomplished with a simple monthly self-examination.

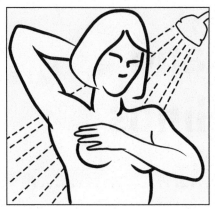
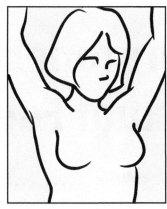
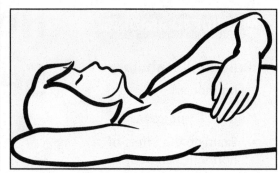

- While taking a shower or bath, gently explore both breast and underarm areas with your fingertips. Check the upper and outer parts of each breast, moving toward the armpit.

- Stand in front of a mirror. Check for changes in size, shape, and contour of each breast. Check for redness, swelling, or changes in the nipple.

- Lie down with one arm tucked behind the head. With the other hand, examine the opposite breast for lumps, thickening, or other changes. Move your fingers around the breast in a circle, then up and down, covering the entire breast area. Repeat on the other breast.

LESSON 2 ASSESSMENT

After You Read
Reviewing Facts and Vocabulary

1. Define the terms *cervix* and *uterus* and explain how these parts of the female reproductive system function.

2. List the external and internal female reproductive organs.

3. Name two disorders of the female reproductive system. Explain why it is important to look for warning signs and seek early detection to prevent disease.

4. Analyze the importance of good personal hygiene for disease prevention. Describe three ways to care for the female reproductive system.

Thinking Critically

5. **Synthesize.** How might you respond if a friend told you she always experiences PMS the week before her menstrual period?

6. **Analyze.** A female who is experiencing symptoms of vaginitis goes to see her doctor. Write a paragraph that suggests how the doctor might be able to distinguish among these possible conditions: a yeast infection, bacterial vaginosis, and trichomoniasis.

Applying Health Skills

7. **Advocacy.** A favorite cousin of yours, who is 22 years old, tells you she has never had a Pap test. She says that seeing a doctor and getting a Pap test aren't important until females are much older. Write your cousin a letter in which you explain what you have learned about regular health care for the female reproductive system.

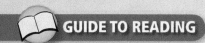

GUIDE TO READING

Building Vocabulary
▸ hormones

Health Concepts
- Examine the effect of hormones on body systems.
- Demonstrate healthful decision-making skills that show responsible behaviors for your health and the health of others.

Reading Strategy
Predict Write a brief paragraph describing what information you believe this lesson will contain.

Hormones and Sexual Feelings

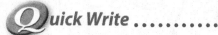

$\mathcal{Q}$uick Write ....

On a sheet of paper, list as many physical changes or reactions as you can think of that are caused by hormones.

Sexual feelings are normal and healthy. They are controlled by the same hormones that affect your physical growth. **Hormones** are *chemical substances produced in glands, which regulate the activities of different body cells and organs*. Sexual feelings are essential for the reproductive process.

Sexual Feelings and Response

Sex hormones cause the body to respond to sexual stimulation, which may result from a kiss, watching a movie scene, holding hands, or thinking about a date. The heart rate increases, breathing speeds up, hands feel clammy, and the face gets flushed. In the male, the penis becomes erect; in the female, vaginal fluids are produced. These are the body's first responses to excitement. They are entirely natural, and people cannot keep them from occurring. However, a person can and must decide what to do about them.

It can become difficult to make a responsible decision once sexual tension builds up. Teens, in particular, can feel overwhelmed by these urges because these feelings are new. The beginning of sexual feelings indicate that you are approaching adulthood. It is a good idea to establish predetermined limits on sexual behavior.

Sexual Feelings and Responsible Decisions

Remember, hormones cause sexual feelings, and sexual feelings are a normal physical response. You have complete control over what you do about these feelings. When they occur, the important thing is to consciously choose to act responsibly.

Health Skills Activity

Goal Setting

Achieving Individual Goals

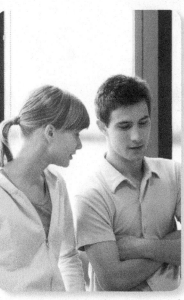

Ray and Shauna have been dating for more than a year. They are concerned about what will happen to them in the future.

"Do you think we'll go to the same college?" Ray asks.

"I don't know," Shauna answers. "I want to study music. You want a career in medical research. I don't think the same school will be right for both of us."

"Well, you could be right, Shauna. But maybe we can find what we want and still be close to each other."

Shauna looks down at her hands and then looks up at her boyfriend. "Oh, Ray. I want to be close to you, too. Do you think we could find good programs in schools that are close so we could still spend time together?"

Ray looks back at Shauna. "We won't know unless we try."

What Would You Do?

Apply the steps of the goal-setting process to Ray and Shauna's situation.

1. Identify a specific goal, and write it down.
2. List the steps you will take to reach that goal.
3. Get help and support from others.
4. Set up checkpoints to evaluate progress.
5. Plan a reward for achieving the goal.

If you feel overwhelmed by sexual feelings, remind yourself of your long-term goals. Engaging in sexual behavior may have consequences that affect your long-term health, and your future. Keeping your goals in mind will help you make mature, responsible decisions.

Remember that your body has some urges that you cannot control. Whether you want to or not, you will sometimes feel hungry, sleepy, or sexually aroused. Just as you can control what you eat and when you sleep, you also control how you respond to sexual feelings. By controlling how you react to sexual arousal, you are taking steps toward behaving maturely and making responsible decisions that will help you to reach your goals for the future and to build a positive self-concept.

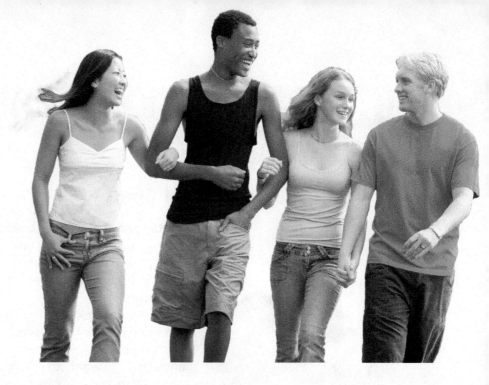

■ **Figure 3.11**
Responsible decisions about sexual feelings are easier to make when shared activities take place that involve lots of other people and interesting things to see and do.

LESSON 3 📖 ASSESSMENT

After You Read

Reviewing Facts and Vocabulary

1. What causes the body's response to sexual stimulation?

2. Name four of the body's first physiological responses to sexual stimulation.

3. Explain why it is important for a teen to establish predetermined limits on sexual behavior before he or she encounters a situation where a decision must be made.

Thinking Critically

4. **Evaluate.** Are sexual feelings and love the same thing? Explain your answer.

5. **Analyze.** Discuss how keeping your long-term goals in mind can help you make mature, responsible decisions when you experience sexual urges. How can these decisions affect your health and the health of others?

Applying Health Skills

6. **Goal Setting.** Identify one of your long-term goals. Draw a cartoon strip in which your focus on this goal helps you and a date choose an activity that you can enjoy together without placing yourself in a sexual situation.

Reviewing Facts and Vocabulary

1. Describe the structure and function of the epididymis.
2. What is the duct that travels through the penis?
3. Describe the composition of semen.
4. What type of movement can cause an inguinal hernia?
5. What are the fallopian tubes, and what role do they play in the female reproductive system?
6. Between what ages do most females begin menstruating?
7. Name three causes of sterility in males. Name three causes of infertility in females.
8. What are three symptoms of breast cancer?

Writing Critically

9. **Evaluate.** Write down some important health decisions you can make to keep your reproductive system healthy.
10. **Synthesize.** Write a one-page summary describing the reproductive process, including how many chromosomes are combined to produce a human offspring.
11. **Synthesize.** Write a summary describing what is unique about the male and female reproductive systems when compared to the other systems of the body.
12. **Analyze.** Write a summary describing how ovulation, menstruation, and fertilization are interrelated.

Applying Health Skills

13. **Advocacy.** Your friend has told you that she has had an unusual vaginal discharge for several days. She is worried and afraid to tell anyone else. Write a dialogue that helps her to overcome her fears and understand how important it is to get medical care so that her condition can be properly identified and treated.
14. **Communication Skills.** A younger sibling of your own gender seems upset. When you ask what is wrong, he or she expresses worry about becoming a teen. Discuss with your younger sibling what to expect during puberty.

Activity Beyond the Classroom

Parent Involvement

School nurse. Invite the school nurse into the classroom to discuss issues concerning puberty and reproductive health. Have parents attend the class session to hear the nurse's presentation. List positive ways that teens can promote their reproductive health.

School and Community

Adolescent health. Interview a health care provider who specializes in adolescent care. Describe the academic preparation necessary for that career and the personal characteristics necessary to be successful in that field.

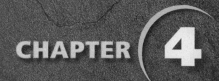

Marriage and Parenthood

Photo Credit: Purestock/SuperStock

Activating Prior Knowledge

Using Visuals Mature, caring adults make good parents. Write three specific responsibilities parents have for their children.

The Commitment to Marry

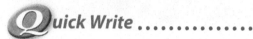

uick Write . . . .

Imagine that your boyfriend or girlfriend has proposed marriage to you. Write a letter to him or her explaining why you are not ready for marriage.

Most people expect to marry during their lifetime. A marriage is different from a dating relationship in many ways. People who enter a marriage make a lifelong commitment to someone they love. A **commitment** is a *promise or a pledge*. In order for a marriage to be successful, both partners must be ready for new responsibilities and challenges. It is very important that couples honestly evaluate themselves, including their goals for the future and for their relationships, in order to determine whether they are ready for the commitment of marriage.

Marriage: A Lifelong Commitment

The most common reason people give for getting married is to enter a lasting relationship with the person they love. Marriage allows couples to share their lives together in an intimate, mature way. It provides companionship in both good and difficult times, in adulthood and into later life.

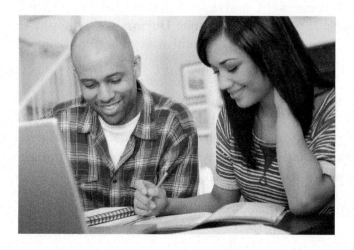

GUIDE TO READING

Building Vocabulary
▶ commitment
▶ blended family

Health Concepts
- Distinguish between a dating relationship and a marital relationship.
- Demonstrate how couples use effective communication skills in building and maintaining healthy relationships.
- Describe the effects of divorce on adults and children.

Reading Strategy
Explain Write a short summary explaining what you think the commitment to marry means. How does committing to marriage change a relationship?

■ **Figure 4.1**
Marriage is a life-changing commitment that requires maturity from both partners. *What can couples do to achieve their goals for the future?*

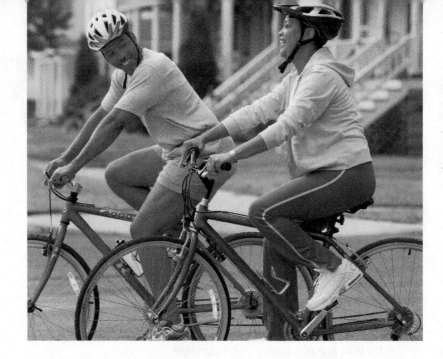

■ **Figure 4.2**

When marriage partners share common interests and activities, their marriage becomes stronger. *Think of a married couple you know and ask how they enjoy their time together.*

Both members of a couple should closely examine their reasons for marrying, and discuss any doubts about marriage. Couples in successful marriages share similar goals and values. Couples considering marriage may want to discuss the following topics:

- How many children does each person want, and when.
- Should the couple marry after completing their education.
- Where will the couple live.
- How will the couple handle conflict.

Adjusting to Marriage

Making a commitment to another person is just the beginning of a successful marriage. Many couples become excited planning a wedding, choosing a place to live together, and sharing their plans with friends and family. They may pay less attention to preparing themselves for marriage. In the early stages of the marriage, couples must face the adjustments that come with marriage—sharing living quarters, finances, and families, for example. During this adjustment period, the emotional and social maturity of both partners is crucial to the success of a marriage.

Mature people understand their own needs as well as their spouse's needs, and they know how to meet those needs in healthy ways. They are willing to compromise and make sacrifices in order to make their marriage successful. Mature couples understand that they will face difficulties in life and that they will work through these difficulties together. Conflicts between a husband and wife will arise, and they will face these challenges with good communication and compassion.

Sociologists have identified a number of factors associated with a successful marriage. In general, a husband and wife should:

- Agree on important issues in their relationship.
- Share common interests and values.
- Demonstrate affection and share confidences.
- Show a willingness to compromise and put others first.
- Share similarities in family backgrounds.
- Have parents who had a successful marriage.
- Not have major conflicts with their in-laws.
- Have several good friends of both genders.
- Have had a long period of close association prior to marriage.
- Have stable jobs and career goals.
- Agree on how they feel about raising children.

Partners with many of these characteristics have an increased chance of building a lasting, happy marriage.

Health Skills Activity

Communication Skills

Expressing Your Feelings to Your Spouse

Tom and Alicia married four months ago. Tom has planned a night out bowling with his friends.

"You're going out again?" Alicia asks, feeling hurt. "I was hoping we could go out to dinner and then have a quiet evening at home."

"I haven't seen the guys in ages," Tom says.

"You just saw them last weekend," Alicia protests. "Our marriage should be more important than bowling night!"

Tom takes a deep breath and wonders what he should do.

What Would You Do?

Use the communication skills you have learned to write an ending to this scenario in which Tom and Alicia express their feelings in productive, nonhurtful ways to resolve their conflict. Be prepared to role-play your response for the class.

1. Use "I" messages.
2. Keep your tone respectful.
3. Provide a clear, organized message that states the problem.
4. Listen to the other person's side without interrupting.

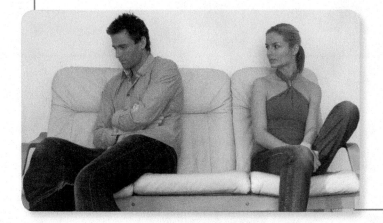

Character Check

Caring If someone you know is going through a difficult divorce, show your compassion and empathy by being available to listen. Make a list of the actions you might take to show your friend that you care.

Marriage and Divorce

Children can be devastated when parents divorce. The family physically separates, and one parent moves out of the home, sometimes to a distant location. Children may feel sad if one parent is not as available to offer guidance. Sometimes children may have to move, which can mean changing schools and leaving friends behind. Families may have to adjust to a lower standard of living because the income is split between two homes. Divorce puts a strain on the entire family and may also impact relationships between individual family members.

In cases where spousal or child abuse is involved, divorce can be a necessary, positive change. Victims of abuse must leave the unsafe environment. Even in situations where there is no abuse, emotional turmoil in the household may create an unhealthy atmosphere for family members. This type of environment can have a permanently negative effect on a child's ability to form healthy relationships later in life. In such cases, divorce may be an appropriate step so that family members can build a new, healthier life.

Although divorce occurs within the marriage of two adults, children may blame themselves for the divorce. Because divorce affects children so strongly, it is essential that parents explore all options, including couples counseling, before making the decision to end the marriage. Above all, both partners should remain responsible parents.

■ Figure 4.3
Seeking help from a professional counselor can help families resolve difficult problems. Even if divorce occurs, counseling can help all family members adjust to the change.

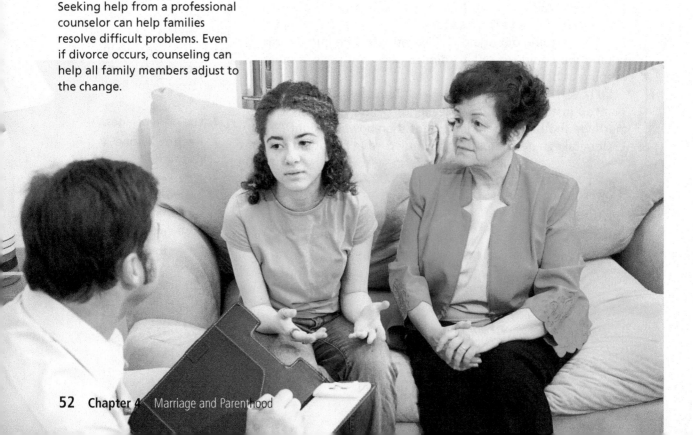

Photo Credit: ©Lisa F. Young/Alamy

Joint Custody

Sometimes divorced couples have joint custody of their children, meaning that the children alternate living with each parent. Depending on work and other schedules, one parent may have the children during the week and the other on weekends, or children may live with one parent for six months of the year and with the other for the rest of the year. Joint custody can create a challenge for the children of a divorced couple. The parents should work together to make the situation less stressful for the children.

Blended Families

People who get divorced may choose to remarry, and it is common for the new spouse to bring his or her own children into the new marriage. This creates a **blended family**, or *a family consisting of two married adults who have children from a previous marriage living with them.* The new couple may also have children together.

Children may experience stress as they adjust to new relationships in the blended family. They may feel resentful of their stepparent or jealous of new stepsiblings. If the stepparent and other children have moved into the child's home, the child may resent having to share it with others. The child may also struggle to get his or her own parent's attention. Emotions such as anger, jealousy, and sadness are normal. To help children adjust to changes after a remarriage, they should be encouraged to talk to their parents, relatives, teachers, counselors, or other trusted adults.

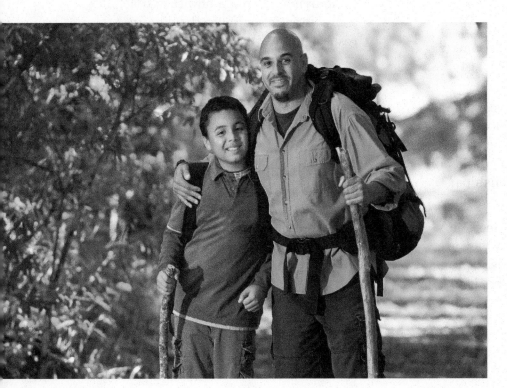

Photo Credit: @iStockphoto.com/goldenKB

■ **Figure 4.4**
Joint custody may be challenging, but it allows both parents to remain involved in their children's lives. *What healthful behaviors can help family members adjust to a divorce?*

Teen Marriage: A Risky Situation

Because a successful marriage requires both people to be responsible and mature, the odds are not in favor of people who marry in their teens. Many teen marriages end in divorce within the first few years.

There are good reasons for teens to delay marriage until they are more mature:

- Married teens have to focus on their spouse's needs and may not have the time or energy to work on their own personal growth and development.

- Married teens may have to postpone college, job training, or beginning a career. With limited earning power, financial difficulties can arise and threaten the marriage.

- If the teen couple married because of a pregnancy, the emotional and financial stresses on the relationship are even more severe.

LESSON 1 ASSESSMENT

After You Read

Reviewing Facts and Vocabulary

1. Define the term *commitment*. How is commitment to a marriage different from commitment to a dating relationship?

2. Explain how a mature couple handles conflict. How does this demonstrate the use of communication skills in building and maintaining healthy relationships?

3. What is a *blended family*?

4. How does making the decision to delay marriage until they are more mature help teens to promote individual and family health?

Thinking Critically

5. Analyze. Describe some characteristics that indicate a couple is ready for marriage. Explain how these characteristics enhance the dignity, respect, and responsibility required in a healthy marriage.

6. Synthesize. Make a list of both positive and negative ways that divorce can affect children.

Applying Health Skills

7. Analyzing Influences. Briefly describe a family sitcom or drama on television. Does the show portray relationships between married couples and their children realistically? How do you think media representations of marriage and family relationships influence viewers?

Photo Credit: ©Ariel Skelley/Blend Images LLC

Becoming a Parent

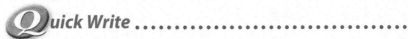

Quick Write . . . .

*Make a word web to describe what you know about caring for an infant. Write the word **Infant** in the middle of a sheet of paper, and circle it. Around the word, write down what responsibilities come to mind. Connect these words and phrases to the center circle.*

Raising children can be the most rewarding and enriching aspect of a person's life. Couples who face the many challenges of parenting feel great joy and love as they watch their children grow. Many married couples find that building a healthy, happy family together is an important, fulfilling life experience.

Why People Have Children

People give all kinds of reasons for having children, including passing on the family name and **heredity**—*genetic characteristics passed from parent to child*—giving one's parents a grandchild, wanting to be loved by someone, giving in to pressure from friends or parents, and bringing stability to a shaky marriage. The only truly good reason for bringing a child into the world is the readiness to raise a family and share the love of the marriage. A new life is a great responsibility, and love for that new life is essential.

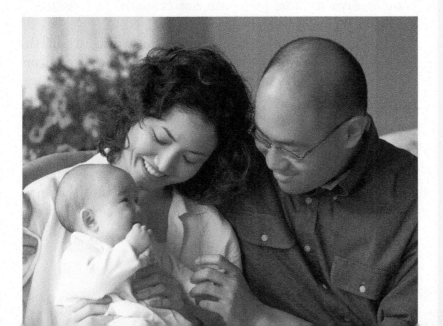

GUIDE TO READING

Building Vocabulary
▸ heredity
▸ parenting
▸ single-parent family

Health Concepts
• Describe the roles and responsibilities of parents.
• Evaluate the effects of family relationships on physical, mental/emotional, and social health.
• Analyze the importance and benefits of abstinence.

Reading Strategy
List Describe some of the responsibilities of parenthood.

■ **Figure 4.5**
Parenting involves nurturing a child's physical, mental/emotional, and social development from infancy through adulthood. *List three specific examples of responsibilities parents have toward their children.*

Lesson 2 Becoming a Parent **55**

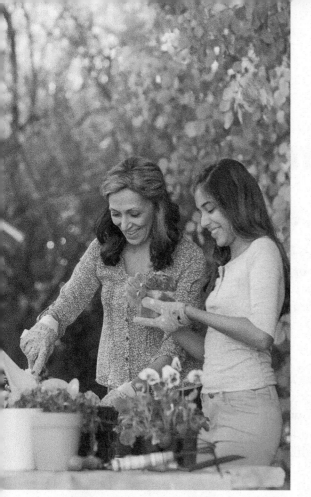

Photo Credit: ©Hero/Corbis/Glow Images

Parental Responsibilities

Parenting, *providing care, support, and love in a way that leads to a child's total development,* is one of the most important jobs anyone can have. Parents must provide the child with basic physical needs: food, clothing, shelter, and medical care. Parents must meet their child's developmental and emotional needs, ensuring that the child is loved unconditionally and receives the proper nurturing and education to prosper later in life.

Parents also need to give guidance to their children, to help them understand right from wrong and develop a good self-concept. By setting limits and providing guidance, parents help children become self-directed and capable of accepting responsibility for their actions. Parents strive to give their children a loving, safe, and supportive environment in which they can grow into responsible, healthy, happy, and independent people.

Parenting skills contribute to strong family relationships. Having this foundation will promote the physical, mental/emotional, and social health of all family members.

■ Figure 4.6
One of the best ways parents can provide a nurturing environment for their children is to spend time with them.

Teen Parenthood

While parenting is rewarding and full of joy, it is also demanding and full of challenges. Even some mature adults may have difficulty adjusting to parenthood. The challenges to teens are even greater.

The reason most teens give for wanting a baby is to have someone who will love them. In the early stages of a child's development, the parent is providing for the child's every need, as well as performing the many tasks associated with the child's care. Parents must be ready to give love, rather than receive it. Most teens are not prepared to handle the demands and responsibilities of raising a child.

Having a baby is tremendously rewarding when the child is brought into a loving, nurturing, and stable environment. However, with all the challenges of adolescence, most teens find the reality of raising a baby to be overwhelming. For most teens, having a baby is not a conscious decision; 78 percent of teen pregnancies are unplanned. A smaller percentage of teens plan to get pregnant, believing that having a child will solve other problems. They quickly find out that the problems have not disappeared and that they now face greater challenges.

Teen parents face many challenges. Some of those challenges include the following:

- Teens may want to escape school or home, only to find they have no support system and a poor career outlook.

- Teens may think that having a baby will strengthen their relationship with their girlfriend or boyfriend. However, having an infant to care for will become the focus of the relationship. This may cause more stress on the relationship of the teen parents.

- Teens may want to prove to themselves or others that they are adults, only to learn how difficult adult responsibilities can be.

- A female teen may want to be the focus of attention, especially while pregnant, but after her baby is born, the infant takes all the attention.

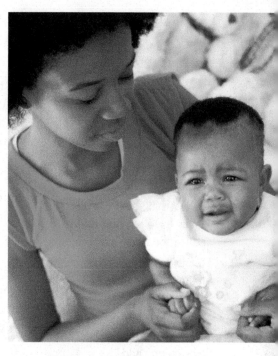

■ **Figure 4.7**
Parenthood brings many responsibilities. The physical, emotional, and financial demands of a new baby can be overwhelming, especially for a teen.

Impact on Physical and Mental/ Emotional Health

Pregnant females require special medical attention to ensure that they stay healthy and have a healthy baby. Regular prenatal care is essential, as is a healthful diet, adequate physical activity and rest, and a strong support network. Teens are the least likely of all age groups to get the proper medical attention, and their diets frequently do not meet the nutritional demands of a growing fetus.

Teen mothers face a higher risk of medical complications, such as early or prolonged labor, high blood pressure, and anemia. For teens younger than 15 years of age, the likelihood of complications is even greater. Babies of teen mothers are more likely to be born with health problems, including those associated with low birth weight. Teens also have more miscarriages.

For a mature adult female, pregnancy can be a joyous, exciting time but also an emotionally stressful one. For a pregnant teen, the stress can become overwhelming because she often does not have the maturity or support she needs.

Impact on Social Health

The around-the-clock demands of a baby make it hard for teen parents to find time and healthy ways to meet their emotional needs. New parents find that their social activities become limited because of their new responsibilities. They often have to juggle difficult schedules and cannot spend time with friends and family as they once did. Their isolation, and their lack of preparation for the parental role, can leave teen parents feeling frustrated and depressed.

Reasons to Wait

These facts explain why teens are not ready to become parents:

- Teens have an increased risk of medical complications while pregnant.

- Teens have not met their educational goals.

- Teens do not have the financial resources to raise a child.

- Teens do not know the developmental needs of a growing child.

■ **Figure 4.8**
Teen fathers face many responsibilities, including providing financially for the child's care.

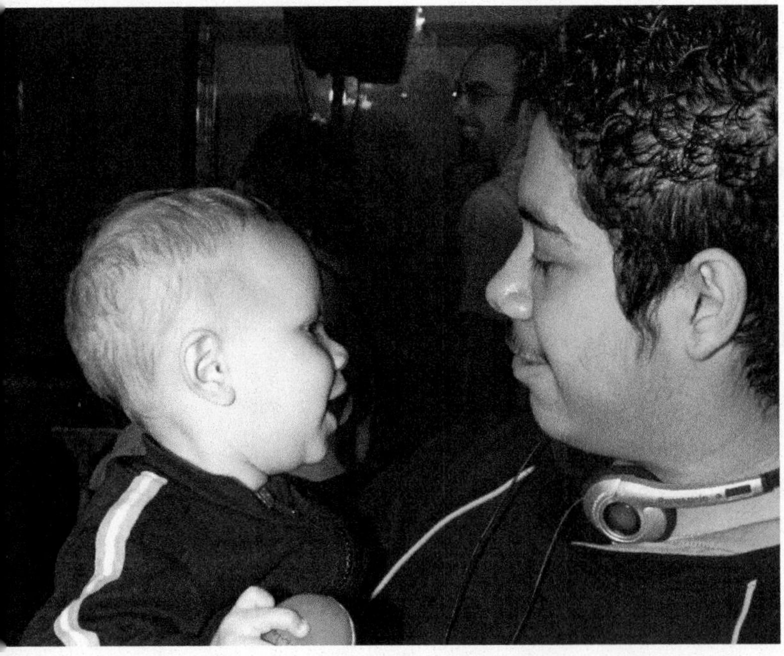

Single Teen Parents

Most female teens who become pregnant do not marry the father of their baby, whether by her choice or his. Even if a teen couple marries, remaining married will be difficult. Most children of teen parents are raised in a **single-parent family**, or *a family that consists of only one parent and one or more children*.

Life for single teen mothers can be difficult. Apart from being less likely to finish high school, teen mothers are dependent on others for financial support, more likely to be poor, and unable to lead the life of a normal teen.

To cope with some of these problems, many teens who are single mothers live with their parents. Some parents can help with child care and provide the financial assistance, love, and support needed by both the mother and her infant. Many states require a teen parent to live with her parents if she is receiving financial aid from the government. If the parents are supportive, living at home is probably the best solution for the teen parents and the child.

Single teen fathers also face difficulties. They often do not have the maturity to provide the child with the necessary care, nurturing, and guidance. In addition, most states require a teen father to provide financial support for his child. A teen father may then have to quit school to get a job. Without a high school diploma, however, he may always have difficulty getting a well-paying job, and college might be beyond reach. Both his emotional and social health may suffer as a result.

Deciding on Teen Parenthood

The decision to delay parenthood until mature and in a committed relationship provides the best opportunity for a happy future. Teen partners should discuss their goals and feelings about the future, and then decide whether they are ready for marriage or children. In a healthy, loving relationship, teen couples support each other's future goals.

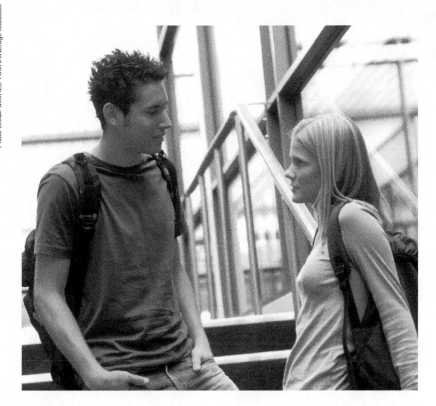

■ Figure 4.9
Couples who choose to remain abstinent can focus on their goals and dreams for the future.

Photo Credit: MICHEL TOURAINE/age fotostock

Responsible teens who are focused on creating a fulfilling future also recognize that abstinence will offer complete protection against pregnancy.

LESSON 2 · ASSESSMENT

After You Read
Reviewing Facts and Vocabulary

1. List reasons people give for deciding to have children.

2. Explain why pregnancy presents a health risk to a teen and her baby.

3. List some of the risks and challenges for a teen father.

Thinking Critically

4. Analyze. Evaluate the effects of parenting and family relationships on physical, mental/emotional, and social health.

5. Evaluate. Describe the roles and responsibilities of parents in promoting healthy families. What do you think are the two most important responsibilities of being a parent? Why?

6. Synthesize. What stressful situations might a teen experience as a result of an unplanned pregnancy? Why is it important for teens to practice abstinence?

Applying Health Skills

7. Refusal Skills. Using information on how pregnancy affects a teen's physical, mental/emotional, and social health, provide ways you could refuse engaging in sexual activity with a boyfriend or girlfriend. Write down at least two specific refusal statements.

Hands-On HEALTH

Activity · Advocating for Abstinence

Committing to abstinence will protect you and your peers from the physical, mental/emotional, and social consequences of teen pregnancy. In this activity, you will create a campaign to increase teen awareness about the importance and benefits of abstinence.

What You'll Need

- Paper and pencils, pens, or markers
- Computer and printer (optional)

What You'll Do

Step 1

In groups of three or four, brainstorm ways to communicate the importance of teen abstinence. Examples may include flyers, posters, newspaper articles, public service announcements, or Web sites. Choose one medium, and develop strategies to carry out your campaign.

Step 2

Analyze the importance and benefits of abstinence. Based on your analysis, create your campaign item and include strong messages about committing to abstinence. Make sure you discuss issues of emotional health and teen pregnancy.

Step 3

Create your campaign, keeping in mind that it should appeal to teens. You might incorporate visual elements, slogans, and attention-getting headlines. Present your completed project to the class.

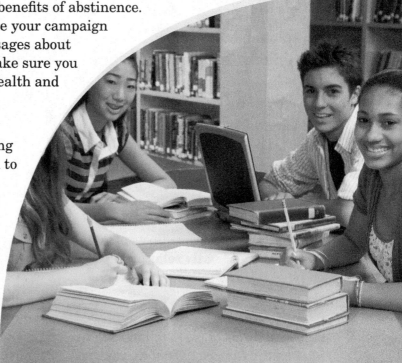

Apply and Conclude

As a class, carry out your campaign in your school or community.

Reviewing Facts and Vocabulary

1. What is the most common reason for people to marry?

2. Describe people who have emotional and social maturity.

3. Identify four factors that can affect marital success.

4. What is *parenting*? Describe the most basic needs a parent provides for a child.

5. How can a female teen's physical health be affected by pregnancy?

6. Name two adjustments a teen male may have to make if he becomes a parent.

7. What is the only sure way to prevent pregnancy until a person is ready to become a parent?

Writing Critically

8. **Analyze.** Write a one-page summary describing what factors should be considered when making the decision to get married.

9. **Synthesize.** Consider the factors that make up a successful marriage, and write down a list of reasons why marriages may end in divorce.

10. **Compare and Contrast.** Make a comparison between a healthy marriage and an unhealthy marriage that you see in the media. Write a list describing what characteristics make up each kind of marriage.

11. **Apply.** Write a brief essay describing what goals you have set for yourself that you would have to delay or give up if you became a teen parent.

12. **Compare and Contrast.** Compare and contrast what it would be like to have a baby as a single teen with what it would be like to have a baby after one is emotionally mature, married, and established in a career. Provide specific examples.

Applying Health Skills

13. **Advocacy.** Create a pamphlet that presents teens with the benefits of remaining abstinent and avoiding teen pregnancy. You can include reasons why being a teen parent is difficult, as well as the actual demands of having and caring for a baby.

14. **Communication Skills.** Write a short story about a teen whose best friend wants to get married and have a baby before finishing high school. The teen should use effective communication skills to discuss with the friend the many risks of teen marriage and pregnancy. Include "I" statements, a respectful and caring tone, and good listening skills.

Activity Beyond the Classroom

Parent Involvement
Research marriage customs. Using the Internet or library resources, find out about marriage customs in the United States. How are they different from the customs of other countries? How are they alike? Discuss these customs with your parents and other family members.

School and Community
Evaluate community resources. Research the amount of money it costs in your community to provide child care for a baby or toddler during a normal 40-hour work week. Find out whether the child care centers provide care for sick children as well. Report your findings to the class.

CHAPTER 5

Pregnancy and Childbirth

Photo Credit: ©Jose Luis Pelaez Inc/Blend Images LLC

Activating Prior Knowledge

Using Visuals A newborn baby's health is greatly affected by the care taken by the mother during pregnancy. What steps can a pregnant female take to ensure that both she and her baby are as healthy as possible?

Prenatal Development

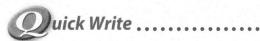uick Write ....

Why is it important to learn about fetal development?
Write down your ideas in a brief paragraph.

Parenthood carries with it the responsibility of providing for a child's physical, mental/emotional, and social well-being. Although physical maturity occurs early in adolescence, mental and emotional maturity that is needed for parenthood generally occurs when adulthood is reached.

Fertilization and Implantation

Pregnancy begins with conception, or **fertilization**—*the union of a single sperm and an ovum.* During sexual intercourse, the erect penis ejaculates hundreds of millions of sperm into the vagina. The sperm swim from the vagina through the cervix, into the uterus, and up the fallopian tubes. If an ovum is present in a fallopian tube, the first sperm that reaches the ovum can penetrate it. *A fertilized ovum* is called a **zygote**. After the zygote forms, it begins dividing, first into two cells, then four, then eight, and so on as it travels down the fallopian tube to the uterus—a journey that takes three to four days. **Figure 5.1** on page 64 illustrates the path of a zygote.

In the uterus, the zygote becomes a **blastocyst**, *a ball of cells with a cavity in the center.* The blastocyst receives nourishment from secretions made by the uterine lining, or endometrium, for another few days before it begins to burrow into, or implant, in the uterine lining.

Embryonic Development

Six or seven days after fertilization, the blastocyst attaches itself to and becomes embedded in the uterine lining, which has been thickening to receive the blastocyst. This process takes a few days. *An implanted blastocyst from the time of*

GUIDE TO READING

Building Vocabulary

▸ fertilization
▸ zygote
▸ blastocyst
▸ embryo
▸ amniotic sac
▸ placenta
▸ umbilical cord
▸ fetus
▸ genes
▸ genetic counseling

Health Concepts

• Explain fetal development from conception through pregnancy.
• Explain the significance of genetics and its role in fetal development.
• Discuss the importance of a healthful lifestyle before and during pregnancy.

Reading Strategy

Predict Scan the headings, subheadings, and photo captions. Write a list of questions related to prenatal development. After reading the lesson, write down the answers to your questions.

Implantation

Fertilization and implantation occur after an egg is released from the ovary.

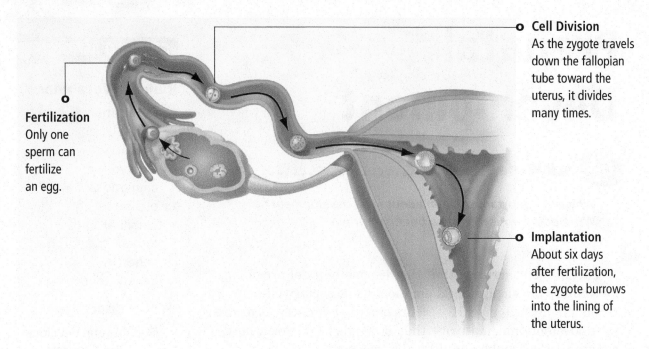

Fertilization
Only one sperm can fertilize an egg.

Cell Division
As the zygote travels down the fallopian tube toward the uterus, it divides many times.

Implantation
About six days after fertilization, the zygote burrows into the lining of the uterus.

Illustration Credit: Linda S. Nye

Why does only one sperm penetrate an ovum?

Immediately after a sperm penetrates an ovum, the ovum's cell membrane undergoes changes that prevent additional sperm from penetrating it. The ovum also releases substances that break down the sperm receptor surrounding the ovum. This makes it impossible for additional sperm to attach to the ovum.

implantation until about the eighth week of development is called an **embryo**. Stages of embryonic development are shown in **Figure 5.3** on page 66.

The embryo grows rapidly during the next five weeks. By the sixth week, it is approximately 4/100 of an inch in size. The cells of the embryo begin to differentiate into three layers that will form the baby's organs and body systems. One layer becomes the respiratory and digestive systems; another develops into muscles, bones, blood vessels, and skin; and a third layer becomes the nervous system, sense organs, and mouth.

One of the first organs to develop is the brain. Neurons begin to develop about 18 days after fertilization. The central nervous system grows rapidly, and the head takes shape about three weeks later.

As development continues, special membranes form around the embryo. One of these membranes becomes the **amniotic sac**, *a fluid-filled sac that surrounds the embryo.* The amniotic sac protects the embryo from outside impact and insulates it from temperature changes. The **placenta** is *a structure that forms along the lining of the uterus as the embryo implants.* The blood-rich tissues of the placenta transfer oxygen and nutrients from the mother's blood to the embryo's blood through the umbilical cord. The **umbilical cord** is *a ropelike structure that connects the embryo and the mother's placenta.* It grows to be about 20 inches long. Waste products leave the embryo's bloodstream through the umbilical cord and are then excreted from the mother's body along with her own wastes.

There is no direct exchange of blood between the mother and the embryo. Materials diffuse from one blood supply to the other through the umbilical cord.

Fetal Development

By the end of the eighth week after fertilization, the major external features of the embryo are formed and the main organ systems are developing. *A developing baby from the end of the eighth week after fertilization until birth* is called a **fetus**. At this point the fetus is only about 1 1/4 inches long, but it is recognizable as a human being. For the remaining 30 weeks of pregnancy, the fetus will continue to grow and develop. See **Figure 5.3** for the stages of fetal development.

Determining a Pregnancy

When fertilization occurs and the blastocyst stage is reached, a hormone called human chorionic gonadotropin (HCG) is released into the mother's bloodstream. This hormone stimulates the release of two other hormones, estrogen and progesterone, which maintain the uterine lining and suppress ovulation. Some HCG passes into the urine. A simple urine test can detect the presence and amount of HCG as early as one day after a missed menstrual period. This confirms whether a female is pregnant. The urine test can be performed at a doctor's office or in the home, using a store-bought pregnancy test.

A radioimmunoassay is another type of pregnancy test that a doctor can perform. This test can detect HCG in urine or blood as early as a week before the expected menstrual period. A doctor will also perform an internal examination to confirm a pregnancy. Changes in the cervix and in the size of the uterus will be detected when a female is pregnant.

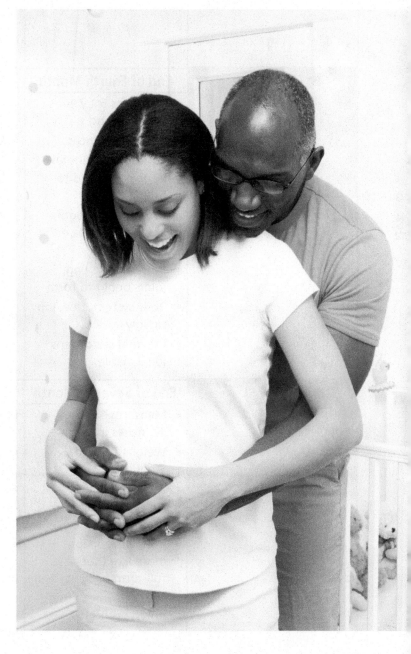

■ **Figure 5.2**
A physician should always confirm the results of a home pregnancy test. *What hormone is detected by pregnancy tests?*

Photo Credit: MedicalRF.com

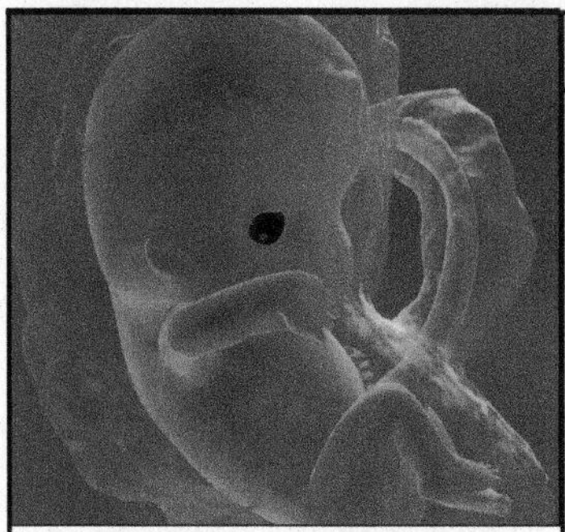

■ Figure 5.3
Stages of Embryonic and Fetal Development

The time from conception to birth is usually about nine full months, which are divided into three 3-month periods called trimesters. This figure describes the changes that take place during each trimester; the images show the development of the fetus in each trimester.

End of First Month	End of Second Month	End of Third Month
• Measures 3/16 of an inch long • Backbone formed • Arm and leg buds begin to form • Heart forms and starts beating	• Measures 1 1/4 inches long • Weighs 1/30 of an ounce • Arms and legs distinguishable, fingers and toes well formed • Eyes visible, eyelids fused • Major blood vessels form • Internal organs continue developing	• Measures 3 inches long • Weighs 1 ounce • Eyes, nose, and ears continue to develop • Heartbeat detectable • Limbs fully formed, nails appear • Urine starts to form
End of Fourth Month	**End of Fifth Month**	**End of Sixth Month**
• Measures 6 1/2 to 7 inches long • Weighs 4 ounces • Head proportionally large compared to body • Face more recognizable, hair forms on head • Bones hardening, joints begin to form • Body systems develop rapidly • External sex organs identifiable	• Measures 10 to 12 inches long • Weighs 1/2 to 1 pound • Lanugo (fine hair) covers body • Fetal movements felt by mother • Head more in proportion with rest of body	• Measures 11 to 14 inches long • Weighs 1 1/4 to 1 1/2 pounds • Eyelids no longer fused, eyelashes form • Skin wrinkled and pink
End of Seventh Month	**End of Eighth Month**	**End of Ninth Month**
• Measures 13 to 17 inches long • Weighs 2 1/2 to 3 pounds • Fetus capable of surviving outside uterus • Body proportions more like that of full-term baby • Fetus assumes upside-down position	• Measures 16 1/2 to 18 inches long • Weighs 4 1/2 to 5 pounds • Fat deposits under skin make skin less wrinkled • In males, testes descend into scrotum • Bones of head soft	• Measures 20 inches long • Weighs 7 to 7 1/2 pounds • Additional fat deposits under skin • Lanugo falls off • Nails fully grown

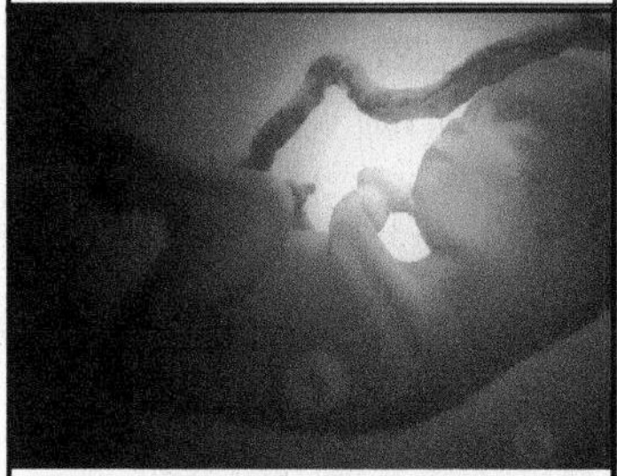

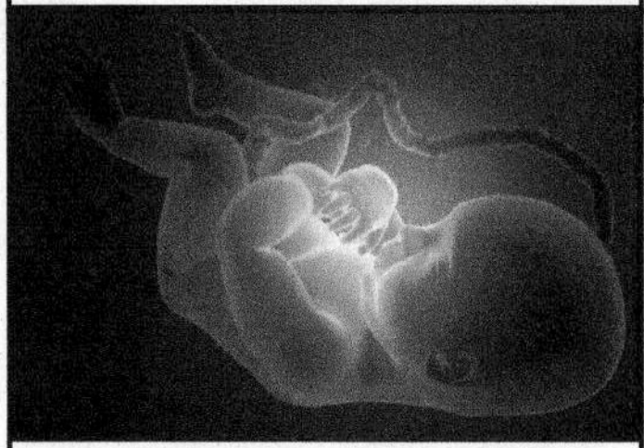

Home pregnancy tests became available in the 1970s. Today, they are the most common form of pregnancy testing. The test is similar to the one given in a doctor's office. However, research has shown that home pregnancy tests yield a high number of false negative results, which means that the test indicates a female is not pregnant when she really is. The unreliability of the test is mostly due to user error; thus, a female should see a physician to confirm the test results.

A Girl or a Boy?

The sperm determines a child's gender. The sperm and the ovum each contribute one set of 23 chromosomes during fertilization. A human being, therefore, has 23 pairs of chromosomes. One pair consists of specialized sex chromosomes, of which there are two types, X and Y. Ova always carry an X (female) chromosome; sperm can carry either an X or a Y. If a sperm carrying an X chromosome fertilizes an ovum, the combination is XX, and the child is female. If the sperm is carrying a Y chromosome, the combination is XY, and the child is male.

Genes and Heredity

The 23 pairs of chromosomes in the human body are made up of genes. **Genes** are *units of heredity that determine which traits, or characteristics, offspring inherit from their parents.* The genes we inherit determine traits such as height, hair color, and skin type.

For some traits, there are two types of genes, dominant and recessive. When both are present in an individual, the dominant gene will mask the effect of the recessive gene. For example, the gene for brown eyes is dominant and the gene for blue eyes is recessive. If a child inherits a gene for blue eyes from each parent, the child will have blue eyes; if a gene for brown eyes comes from each parent, the child's eyes will be brown. However, if a child inherits a gene for brown eyes from one parent and a gene for blue eyes from the other parent, the dominant gene for brown eyes will mask the effect of the recessive gene for blue eyes, and the child will have brown eyes.

Hereditary Diseases

Certain diseases can be passed from parent to offspring through genes. The genes for some hereditary diseases are dominant; thus, only one parent has to contribute that gene for the child to have the disease. Some genetic diseases can be recognized in the womb. These tests are usually done when a pregnancy is confirmed.

If a parent has this incurable disease, there is a fifty percent chance that he or she will pass the disease on to the child. In hereditary diseases for which the gene is recessive, both parents must contribute the gene for their child to have the disease. Parents can carry a recessive gene for the disease without having the disease themselves if they have a dominant gene to mask it. Cystic fibrosis is a recessive gene disorder. In this fatal disease, the body produces abnormally thick and sticky mucus in the lungs and other parts of the respiratory system.

Certain recessive gene diseases are carried only on the X chromosome. Because a female has two X chromosomes, she can have one dominant and one recessive gene and not have the disease. Because males have only one X chromosome, if they inherit a recessive gene for the disease, there is no paired dominant gene to mask it. Hemophilia and red-green color blindness are examples of this type of genetic disease.

Genetic Counseling

Genetics is the study of heredity. **Genetic counseling** is *a process in which genetic histories of prospective parents are studied to determine the presence of certain hereditary diseases.* People's family histories can be mapped, and medical tests can be run to identify genetic or biochemical markers for certain hereditary diseases, such as Huntington's disease. Since most people don't show symptoms of this disease until later in life, genetic testing before pregnancy can help married couples make an informed decision about having children.

LESSON 1   ASSESSMENT

After You Read
Reviewing Facts and Vocabulary

1. List and briefly explain the major steps of fetal development from conception to birth.

2. Describe the function of the amniotic sac.

3. What will a doctor do to determine if a female is pregnant?

4. Does the father's sperm or the mother's ovum determine a child's gender? How?

5. What are *genes*? List some characteristics that are inherited.

Thinking Critically

6. Synthesize. If a child has one parent with brown eyes and one parent with blue eyes, what color eyes will the child have? Why?

7. Analyze. In a short paragraph, briefly explain the significance of genetics and its role in fetal development.

Applying Health Skills

8. Communication Skills. Suppose a friend tells you she is not pregnant because she took a home pregnancy test and the results were negative. What would you tell her?

Prenatal Care

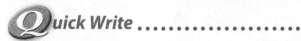 **Q**uick Write ....

List three things a pregnant female should do and three things she should not do to ensure the health of her baby.

Early signs of pregnancy vary. Some signs such as food cravings, headaches, swollen/tender breasts, and spotting or cramping may be mistaken for the start of a menstrual period. Early testing is important because the sooner a pregnancy is confirmed, the sooner prenatal care can begin. **Prenatal** means *occurring or existing before birth*. Prenatal care increases the odds of a healthy pregnancy. As soon as a female knows she is pregnant, she should seek prenatal care.

Characteristics of a Pregnancy

A normal pregnancy lasts about nine full months. Pregnancy can be divided into three trimesters, or periods of three months, each characterized by physical changes and symptoms:

- **First Trimester.** The breasts become fuller and tender, and blood vessels in the breasts become more prominent. The areola, the area around each nipple, darkens. Many females experience morning sickness—nausea or vomiting that occurs most frequently in the morning—and even mild exertion may bring on fatigue.

- **Second Trimester.** The fetus continues to grow, causing the abdomen to swell; the mother can detect fetal movements. Both appetite and blood volume increase. Morning sickness usually subsides, and many females report feeling healthy and energetic during this time.

- **Third Trimester.** Pregnancy is almost always visible by the third trimester. Most females will have gained 25 to 35 pounds by the time of delivery. Blood volume has increased by 30 to 40 percent, the mother's heart beats faster, and the uterus is stretched to many times its original size. After the birth, the uterus contracts to nearly its pre-pregnancy size. The growing fetus takes up enough room to crowd the mother's bladder, stomach, and lungs.

Building Vocabulary

- prenatal
- fetal alcohol syndrome (FAS)
- rubella
- ultrasound
- amniocentesis
- chorionic villi sampling (CVS)
- birth defect

Health Concepts

- Analyze how alcohol, tobacco, and other drugs affect the fetus.
- Explain the importance of prenatal care and proper nutrition for the baby and mother.
- Explain how technology has impacted families by aiding in prenatal diagnosis of certain conditions.

Reading Strategy

Explain Write a summary describing what the term *prenatal care* means. What behaviors might a mother change to take care of her baby before it is born?

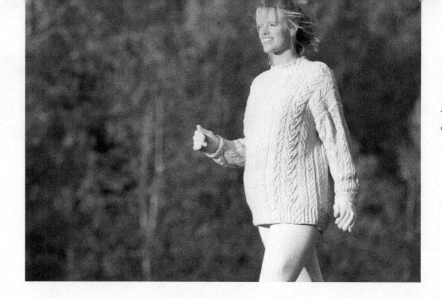

Photo Credit: Getty Images

■ **Figure 5.4**
During the second trimester, most pregnant females feel healthy and energetic. *How long does a normal pregnancy last?*

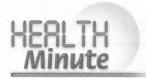

Physical Activity Recommendations

Regular physical activity during pregnancy helps:

• **Prevent unnecessary weight gain.**

• **Increase blood circulation.**

• **Reduce fatigue and improve sleep.**

• **Prepare the mother for the rigors of labor.**

• **Improve mental health and well-being.**

Mental/Emotional Changes

Hormonal changes cause many pregnant females to become more emotional or experience mood swings similar to those associated with premenstrual syndrome (PMS). In the first trimester, feelings can range from joy to fear to excitement. In the second trimester, hormonal shifts may cause forgetfulness. Some females may also have difficulty concentrating. As a pregnant female gains weight, her center of gravity changes and her ligaments loosen; this may cause her to feel more clumsy than usual. In the third trimester, worries about labor, delivery, and the health of the baby are all normal. Talking about these feelings with a caring partner, a physician, or another pregnant female can be helpful.

Common Discomforts

The growing fetus causes changes in a female's body that can bring on a range of discomforts during pregnancy. The need to urinate increases, and many females experience leg cramps. Headaches, particularly in the first trimester, are also common. In the later months, back pain can result from increased weight in the front, and water retention causes swelling of the hands, ankles, and feet. Minor contractions and sleep problems may occur. Weight gain can result in the development of stretch marks, which a pregnant female may find unsightly. With the exception of stretch marks, these discomforts usually end after delivery.

Components of Prenatal Care

The care a female takes during pregnancy affects her own health, as well as that of her developing baby. Regular medical care, a well-balanced eating plan, regular physical activity, and avoidance of harmful substances such as tobacco, alcohol, and other drugs are all responsible choices that a pregnant female can make.

Medical Care

The main component of prenatal care is a schedule of regular visits with an obstetrician or certified nurse-midwife. Both types of health care providers are trained in prenatal care and delivery of babies. The obstetrician or nurse-midwife takes a medical history and gives the pregnant female a complete physical examination, which includes blood and urine tests as well as a pelvic examination. Regular visits are usually scheduled once a month through the seventh month, every two weeks in the eighth month, and weekly in the ninth month. At each visit, the mother's weight and blood pressure will be taken, her urine tested, her abdomen measured, and (from week 12) the fetal heartbeat monitored.

Nutrition and Physical Activity

A pregnant female needs to consume more nutrients to ensure the health of the developing fetus. She needs extra protein for her own strength and for the development of the placenta, amniotic sac, and fetal brain. She needs extra calcium to build strong fetal bones and teeth, vitamin E for tissue growth and red blood cells, and iron for red blood cells. Inadequate iron intake can lead to fatigue and possibly anemia. Doctors recommend that all pregnant females take prenatal vitamins to ensure that they are getting adequate nutrients.

Another necessary nutrient is folic acid. This B vitamin is a critical part of spinal fluid and helps close the tube that contains the central nervous system. This neural tube forms 17 to 30 days after conception, so neural tube defects can occur before a female knows that she is pregnant. Health care professionals suggest that all females of childbearing age consume 400 to 600 micrograms of folic acid daily to prevent neural tube defects.

For females who are at a healthy pre-pregnancy weight, gaining more than 35 pounds during pregnancy can be a health risk for both mother and baby. Daily caloric intake should increase by only about 300 calories, and those additional calories should come from nutritious foods, including those rich in calcium and protein.

Physical activity is important during pregnancy. In a normal pregnancy, most activities a healthy female participated in before she became pregnant can be continued. Walking and swimming are particularly good activities during pregnancy.

Medical Complications

In a normal pregnancy, there are no major problems. Proper prenatal care can help identify and treat medical complications when they do arise.

■ **Figure 5.5**
Good nutrition ensures that a pregnant female receives the nutrients required for proper fetal development.

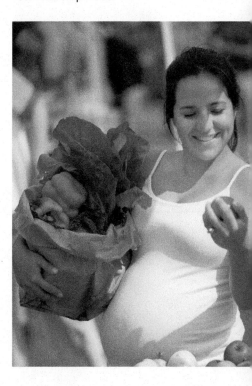

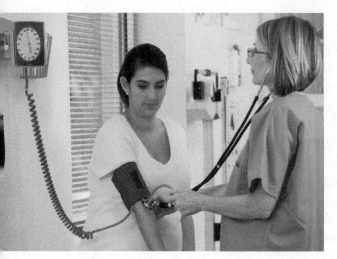

■ **Figure 5.6**
Regular prenatal checkups can help identify potential complications during pregnancy. *Why is it important for a pregnant female to have her blood pressure checked regularly?*

Rh Factor in Blood. Rh factor is a protein on the surface of red blood cells. About 85 percent of people have this antigen in their blood and are called Rh+ (Rh positive). Those who do not have it are Rh– (Rh negative). When an Rh– person receives Rh+ blood, their blood builds up antibodies against the Rh antigen. If an Rh– mother and an Rh+ father have an Rh+ baby, the mother's antibodies can cross the placenta and attack the baby's red blood cells. Treatment of the mother with a serum known as Rh immune globulin can prevent the buildup of antibodies, but the problem must be diagnosed early to avoid serious fetal complications.

Pregnancy-Induced Hypertension and Preeclampsia. The mother's blood pressure normally rises a bit around the seventh month, but about 5 to 10 percent of pregnant females develop prolonged high blood pressure, or pregnancy-induced hypertension (PIH).

If PIH is accompanied by sudden weight gain, severe swelling from water retention, and/or protein in the urine, the female has a condition known as preeclampsia. If untreated, this condition can lead to many health problems for the mother, ranging from blurred vision and headaches to convulsions and coma. Preeclampsia can also cause stunted growth and mental retardation in the fetus. First-time mothers in their early teens or those over age 35 are most at risk. Complete bed rest and medication can increase the chances of a full-term delivery, but sometimes the baby must be delivered early to protect both mother and baby.

Dangers to the Fetus

Although mother and baby do not directly share any blood, substances in the mother's bloodstream cross the placenta and enter the fetus's blood. No medication should be taken without a physician's advice, and alcohol, tobacco, and illegal drugs should be avoided entirely.

Tobacco. Tobacco use is harmful to both mother and baby. Babies born to females who smoke can have lower birth weights, heart and brain abnormalities, and cleft lips and palates. Smoking has been linked to higher fetal and infant mortality rates, as well as sudden infant death syndrome (SIDS), a condition in which a seemingly healthy baby dies for no apparent reason. Secondhand smoke also poses a health risk, according to the American Lung Association, which states that pregnant females exposed repeatedly to secondhand smoke have an increased risk of having a low birth-weight baby.

Alcohol. Fetal alcohol syndrome (FAS) is *a condition of physical, mental, and behavioral abnormalities that can result when a pregnant female drinks alcohol.* Effects on the fetus include low birth weight, general weakness, impaired speech, poor coordination, stunted growth, cleft palate, facial and heart defects, mental retardation, poor attention span, inability to understand the consequences of actions, and hyperactivity. Fetal alcohol syndrome cannot occur unless alcohol is consumed. The safest decision for pregnant females and those considering pregnancy is not to drink any alcoholic beverages.

Medications and Drugs. All medications and supplements must be approved for use during pregnancy by a health care professional. This includes prescription and over-the-counter products, as well as those labeled "natural" or "herbal." Many seemingly safe substances can harm the fetus.

All illegal drugs are unsafe and can cause serious health problems in the fetus, including mental retardation, respiratory problems, visual and hearing disabilities, learning and emotional problems, low birth weight, and even death. A baby can also be born addicted to a drug and have to go through the painful and dangerous process of withdrawal.

Caffeine. Some studies suggest that consuming caffeinated products during pregnancy may pose health risks to the fetus. Coffee, tea, chocolate, cola drinks, and certain other soft drinks may contain caffeine. Many females choose to avoid caffeine during pregnancy to help ensure their baby's health.

Rubella. Rubella (German measles) is *a contagious disease caused by a virus that does not cause serious complications except in pregnancy.* Symptoms include a rash, swollen glands, and joint pain, particularly in adults. Most pregnant females are immune to the disease either through vaccination or because they had the disease as children. Nevertheless, about 20 percent of females of childbearing age are not immune to rubella. If a pregnant female contracts rubella, especially during the first trimester, her fetus may develop severe birth defects. These include vision and hearing loss, heart defects, and mental retardation. Rubella infection can cause miscarriage, which is the spontaneous expulsion of a fetus before the twentieth week of pregnancy. It may also cause stillbirth, the expulsion of a dead fetus from the body after the twentieth week of pregnancy. If a female contracts rubella after 20 weeks of pregnancy, birth defects are rare.

Other Dangers. Direct exposure to radiation can harm a developing fetus, so it is best to avoid routine X-rays such as those taken by a dentist. If X-rays are necessary, however, as in the case of a broken bone, a protective apron can be placed over the abdomen to shield it from radiation.

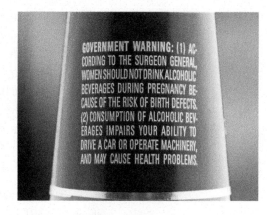

■ **Figure 5.7**
Alcohol consumption during pregnancy can cause many serious health problems in the fetus.

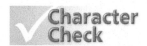
Character Check

Responsibility Pregnant females have a responsibility to protect the developing fetus by avoiding the use of harmful substances such as tobacco, alcohol, and other drugs.
Create a pamphlet explaining why it is especially important for a female to avoid using harmful substances during pregnancy.

Maternal exposure to lead can also endanger a fetus, causing developmental defects and mental deficiency when lead in the mother's bloodstream passes through the placenta to the fetus's blood. One common source of lead is paint in buildings built before 1978, when lead-based paint was banned. Maternal lead exposure can also cause higher rates of miscarriage, premature birth, and stillbirth.

Sexually Transmitted Diseases

Sexually transmitted diseases (STDs) are diseases spread through sexual contact; some are very harmful to a fetus and newborn (see **Figure 5.8**). Because of the serious threat posed by STDs, pregnant females are tested for these diseases at the first prenatal visit with their health care professional. Some STDs can be cured, but others can be only treated. Females who know they have an STD should seek treatment before they become pregnant.

Tests During Pregnancy

Prenatal tests may be ordered to see if a fetus is at risk for various health problems. Sometimes a problem can be treated before the baby is born.

■ **Figure 5.8**

Effects of STDs on the Fetus and Infant

STD	Time of Transmission	Harm to Fetus/Infant	Treatment
Chlamydia	During delivery	Premature delivery, eye and respiratory infections, blindness, pneumonia	Antibiotics
Gonorrhea	During delivery	Blindness, joint infections, blood infections	Antibiotics
Herpes	During delivery	Fatal infections, lesions on eyes or mouth	No cure; antiviral medications can minimize outbreaks; cesarean delivery can protect the baby
Human papillomavirus (HPV)	During delivery	Development of warts in throat or voice box	No cure; surgery to prevent warts from blocking throat
Syphilis	During pregnancy	Stillbirth, developmental delays, seizures, death shortly after birth	Intramuscular injection of antibiotic
HIV	During pregnancy/ delivery/breastfeeding	Weak immune system, thrush, bacterial infections, neurological problems, enlarged lymph nodes, liver, and spleen	No cure; AZT helps prevent transmission from mother to child

Ultrasound

The fetus can be seen in the uterus by using **ultrasound**, *a test that produces an image on a screen by reflecting sound waves off the body's inner structures.* The embryo is visible by four weeks after fertilization, and the fetal heartbeat can be identified at five weeks. To produce an image, an instrument called a transducer is moved across the abdomen; a computer translates the reflections into images on a monitor. Ultrasound can be used throughout pregnancy to assess fetal position and development.

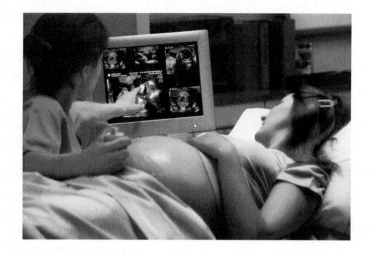

Photo Credit: ©Jose Luis Pelaez Inc/Blend Images LLC

Figure 5.9
An ultrasound allows a fetus to be observed without exposing either the mother or the fetus to the radioactivity of X-rays.

Amniocentesis

Amniocentesis is *a procedure that reveals chromosomal abnormalities and certain metabolic disorders in the fetus.* First, ultrasound is used to determine the position of the fetus. The doctor then inserts a long needle through the abdomen and into the amniotic sac and removes 1 to 2 tablespoons of amniotic fluid. The fluid contains living cells from the fetus that are tested for chromosomal abnormalities and also reveal the gender and age of the fetus. Amniocentesis is usually performed 16 to 20 weeks after fertilization. The procedure carries a small risk of miscarriage. Because of this risk, amniocentesis is usually recommended only for those females who have an increased risk of having a child with chromosomal or genetic abnormalities. Factors that may contribute to these abnormalities include the following:

- The mother is 35 years of age or older.
- The mother has had a previous child or fetus with a birth defect.
- There is a family history of certain chromosomal or genetic disorders.

Chorionic Villi Sampling

In addition to amniocentesis, *a test used to reveal genetic disorders and fetal age and gender* is **chorionic villi sampling** (CVS). In this procedure, a thin tube is inserted through the vagina and the cervix. A small sample of chorionic villi, tissue attached to the sac that contains the fetus, is removed. The test is usually done between 10 and 12 weeks after a female's last menstrual period; results are available within 10 days. CVS is slightly more likely than amniocentesis to cause miscarriage.

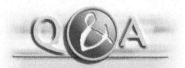

How does amniocentesis enable doctors to learn a fetus's gender?

The living fetal cells in the amniotic fluid removed during amniocentesis are cultured, or grown in a laboratory. During the subsequent analysis of the chromosomes for abnormalities, the chromosomes are paired and identified. The pairing of sex chromosomes indicates the sex of the fetus—XX for a female, XY for a male.

Like amniocentesis, CVS is usually offered only to pregnant females who have an increased risk of giving birth to a child with genetic or chromosomal abnormalities. Some parents choose CVS because the test can be performed earlier than amniocentesis.

Birth Defects

A **birth defect** is *an abnormality in the structure or function of the body that is present at birth. Birth defects can be caused by abnormal genes or by environmental factors.* About one in every 33 infants are born with a birth defect. There are more than 4,000 known birth defects. Environmental factors that may cause birth defects include maternal exposure to toxins, maternal diseases, and maternal substance abuse. They also include problems that may arise during delivery, such as when the fetus does not receive an adequate supply of oxygen. Many physical defects, such as cleft lip and clubfoot, are visible at birth. Mental defects such as retardation, cerebral palsy, and brain dysfunction may not be observed until the child is older. Other conditions that are present at birth may not be apparent until the child is several months to a year old, or even older. Sickle-cell anemia and cystic fibrosis are examples of such defects.

LESSON 2 ASSESSMENT

After You Read
Reviewing Facts and Vocabulary

1. List two physical changes that occur during each trimester.

2. How can alcohol, tobacco, other drugs, and environmental hazards harm a fetus?

3. What is *fetal alcohol syndrome*?

4. Name two tests that can be done during pregnancy to see if the baby is at risk for a genetic or chromosomal abnormality.

Thinking Critically

5. Synthesize. Explain the importance of the role of prenatal care and proper nutrition in promoting optimal health for both the baby and the mother.

6. Analyze. Briefly explain how technology has impacted the health status of families by aiding in prenatal diagnosis of certain conditions.

Applying Health Skills

7. Refusal Skills. Suppose you have an older sister who is pregnant. Some of her friends are trying to convince her that it's okay to drink alcohol during her pregnancy. Explain to her why she needs to use refusal skills, and suggest ways to say no effectively.

Childbirth

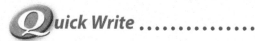

Briefly explain why a pregnant female needs to have regular exams by a health care professional.

At the end of the pregnancy, the hormone oxytocin causes uterine contractions that begin to pull open the cervix. This is the beginning of the birthing process.

Stages of Labor

Labor is *the process by which contractions gradually push the baby out of the uterus and into the vagina to be born.* Though each female's pregnancy and delivery is unique, it is important to understand the typical stages leading up to labor. Labor has three stages:

- **First Stage of Labor.** Contractions gradually open the cervix to a diameter of about four inches. This process of dilation is the first, and usually longest, stage of labor. The amniotic sac is a membrane filled with fluid that cushions the baby as it develops. The pressure of the baby's head against the amniotic sac during this stage or the next usually causes the sac to rupture, or the pregnant female's water to "break." About a pint of amniotic fluid is released from the vagina. The first stage may last for 12 hours or longer.

- **Second Stage of Labor.** When the cervix is fully dilated, the mother feels an urge to push. She uses muscles to aid the contractions in pushing the baby's head through the cervix and into the vagina.

   When the baby's head crowns, or is visible at the vaginal opening, the mother continues pushing until the baby is delivered. This stage generally lasts from 1/2 hour to 2 hours. Rather than risk tearing the tissues around the vaginal opening, a doctor will sometimes perform an **episiotomy**, *an incision made from the vagina toward the anus to enlarge the opening for delivery of a baby.* The incision is stitched back together after the birth.

GUIDE TO READING

Building Vocabulary
- labor
- episiotomy
- cesarean birth
- birthing centers

Health Concepts
- Identify and explain the stages of labor.
- Explain how breast-feeding promotes optimal health for the baby.
- Identify childbirth options and trends.

Reading Strategy
Organize Information
Create a chart listing the stages of labor. Under each section, describe what happens during that stage.

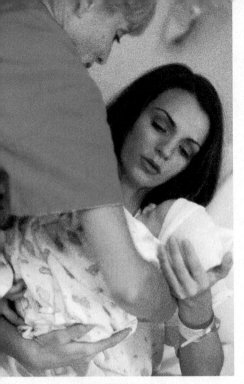

■ Figure 5.10
After a baby is delivered, the doctor or nurse-midwife places the child in the mother's arms.

Photo Credit: Francisco Cruz/Purestock/SuperStock

What is a breech birth?

A breech birth is a birth in which the baby enters the vagina with the buttocks or feet first. The dangers of a breech birth are related to the fact that the baby's head is delivered last. Because the umbilical cord precedes the head, the cord can become compressed when the head moves through the birth canal, cutting off the baby's supply of oxygen. As the head moves quickly through the birth canal, the sudden change in pressure on the skull can result in brain hemorrhage, causing brain damage.

- **Third Stage of Labor.** The final stage of labor lasts about 20 minutes. Contractions separate the placenta or after-birth from the uterine wall and expel the placenta from the uterus and out of the body through the vagina. The detached placenta is called the afterbirth.

Delivery by Cesarean

Cesarean birth is *a method of childbirth in which a surgical incision is made through the abdominal wall and uterus. The baby is lifted out through the surgical incision.* The incidence of cesarean birth, also called cesarean section (C-section) accounting for more than 21 percent of U.S. births in 2012. Some C-sections are performed because the baby is not positioned correctly or does not progress into the vagina, or because the mother's pelvic structure makes a vaginal delivery dangerous or even impossible. C-sections are also used to avoid transmission of certain STDs to the baby as it passes through the vagina. A pregnant female should discuss her views on C-section with her health care provider before labor begins.

Medication During Labor

Some females deliver their babies without pain medication. For those who need pain relief, several medications can be used. Some females find that pain medication relaxes them and helps them deal with the contractions. Others find that the drugs make them too drowsy to concentrate and participate fully in the birth. The effect of pain medications on the baby depends on the amount administered and how close to delivery the drug is given to the mother. If, for example, medications are given shortly before birth, the baby may be drowsy or have difficulty breathing.

When total pain relief is needed, an epidural block is used. Medication injected through a tube inserted between the vertebrae into the spine provides total numbness from the waist down. Epidurals are used during C-sections and some vaginal births. General anesthesia, where the female is unconscious, is used almost exclusively for high-risk cesarean births.

After Delivery

Nursing can begin as soon as the baby is born. While the mother is not yet producing milk, her breasts secrete colostrum, a low-fat, high-carbohydrate, protein-rich fluid. Colostrum is easy to digest and has a laxative effect on the newborn.

After a few days, the breasts begin to produce milk. Both colostrum and milk contain antibodies from the mother; therefore, breast-fed babies get fewer illnesses than babies who are not breast-fed. Breast milk is nutritionally ideal for almost all babies, it doesn't cost anything, it's easier to digest than formula, and it's always ready. Babies aren't allergic to breast milk, but many are allergic to formulas based on cow's milk or soy protein. For these reasons, most pediatricians recommend breast milk over formula.

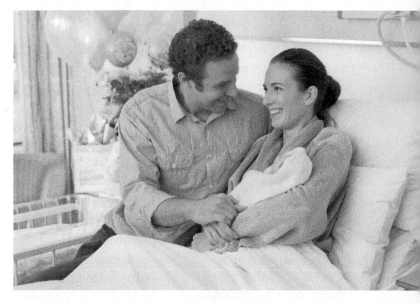

■ **Figure 5.11**
Birthing rooms are designed so that a female can remain in the same hospital room for labor, delivery, and recovery.

Real World **CONNECTION**

Health Information in the News

Recently, news organizations noted an interesting and significant trend in teen pregnancies in the United States, based on statistics from the National Center for Health Statistics. The graph below reflects some of these statistics for pregnancies among females 15 to 19 years of age from 1940 to 2011.

Number of Pregnancies in Females 15-19 Years of Age

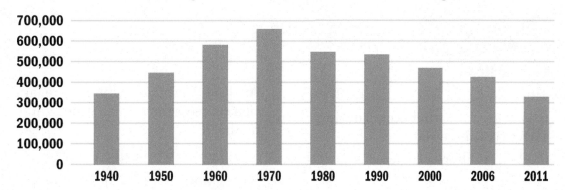

Activity Work in groups of two or three to answer the following questions: How would you describe the overall trend(s) since 1940? In which year were pregnancies highest among this age group? Approximately what percentage decrease occurred between 1970 and 2011? If the trend continues, approximately what number would you expect to see in 2020? Discuss possible reasons for the decline of the last three decades. Be prepared to present your findings to the class.

Photo Credit: ©Chris Ryan/age fotostock

Childbirth: Options and Trends

Many parents choose to educate themselves about the process of childbirth. They attend classes in birthing methods such as Lamaze or Bradley. Most doctors and nurse-midwives recommend that expectant parents attend some type of childbirth classes to learn what to expect at each stage of labor and delivery. The father, a close friend, or a relative learns to play the role of coach; the mother learns relaxation and breathing techniques that enable her to cope with the pain of labor and perhaps have a medication-free delivery. The goal is to make the experience less mysterious and as painless as possible.

Another choice parents can make is where to have their baby. A popular option today is **birthing centers**, *facilities that have homelike settings, are separate from a hospital, and offer medication-free births*. In hospital maternity wards, nurses and doctors deliver the baby, but birthing centers are staffed by certified midwives. Midwives are not registered nurses, but receive training specifically for childbirth. Birthing centers are not designed to handle emergencies and are usually available only for low-risk pregnancies. Because of this, midwives do not perform cesarean sections. However, birthing centers are often located near a hospital in case an emergency does arise. Many hospitals now have their own in-house birthing centers.

LESSON 3 ASSESSMENT

After You Read

Reviewing Facts and Vocabulary

1. Briefly describe what occurs during each of the three stages of labor.

2. Explain what an *episiotomy* is and why it is used.

3. What is a *cesarean birth*?

4. When parents attend classes in birthing methods, what is the goal?

Thinking Critically

5. **Synthesize.** Explain how breast-feeding promotes optimal health for the baby.

6. **Analyze.** How is a childbirth preparation course helpful to an expectant mother?

Applying Health Skills

7. **Stress Management.** In addition to helping a pregnant female prepare for childbirth, classes in birthing methods also teach the expectant mother how to relax. Why might stress interfere with labor and delivery? What are some stress-management techniques a female could use throughout her pregnancy?

Reviewing Facts and Vocabulary

1. What is *fertilization*? How is it related to pregnancy?

2. When is the developing fetus's heartbeat detectable?

3. What happens during genetic counseling?

4. Describe the physical and mental/emotional changes a female may experience during her second trimester of pregnancy.

5. How can tobacco use affect a developing baby?

6. List one reason why a pregnant female would have an ultrasound.

7. About how many known birth defects are there? What can cause them?

8. Describe the second stage of labor.

9. What is taught in childbirth preparation classes?

10. What is a *birthing center*?

Writing Critically

11. **Synthesize.** Write a paragraph describing how the placenta and umbilical cord are integral to the nourishment of the embryo and fetus.

12. **Analyze.** A pregnant female experiences a sudden weight gain. She visits her doctor, who finds that her blood pressure is very high. Write a brief summary describing what condition the doctor would likely suspect. What other symptoms will the doctor check for? Explain your answers.

13. **Analyze.** Write a brief summary explaining why a doctor might recommend a cesarean birth instead of allowing labor and delivery to progress naturally.

Applying Health Skills

14. **Advocacy.** Create a pamphlet that encourages females to seek medical care when they are pregnant. List the reasons why medical care is important throughout the pregnancy as well as during labor and delivery. Make your pamphlet as attractive and informative as possible.

15. **Practicing Healthful Behaviors.** Review the information presented in this chapter. Talk with a pair of prospective parents. Discuss with them what you have learned about healthful behaviors during pregnancy and the birth process.

Activity Beyond the Classroom

Parent Involvement

Medication options. Do research at the library or on the Internet to learn more about the pros and cons of using various medications during labor and delivery. Discuss this issue with your parents or guardians and ask what their views are on the subject.

School and Community

Treatment options. Research the symptoms of postpartum depression at the school or community library. Identify ways that these symptoms can be treated. Present your findings to the class.

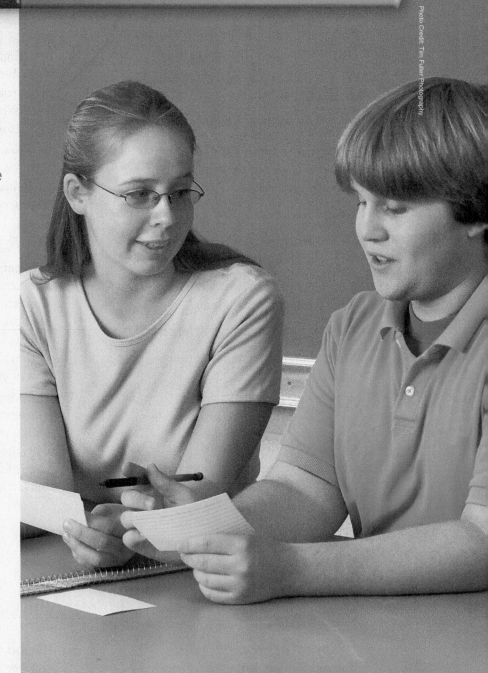

Photo Credit: Tim Fuller Photography

Activating Prior Knowledge

Using Visuals How might having the correct information on sexuality benefit teens? Explain in a paragraph one situation in which having the facts would be important.

Contraception

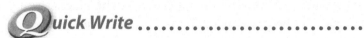

Quick Write ....

> *How much do you know about contraception and STD prevention? Write down three contraceptive methods that you believe also offer protection against STDs.*

In the United States, in 2011, more than 320,000 teens became pregnant. Most of these pregnancies are unplanned. Factors such as lack of correct information, belief of incorrect information, alcohol and drug use, negative peer pressure, and portrayals of risk-free sex in the media all contribute to this serious but preventable problem.

Facts About Pregnancy Prevention

Whenever sperm are in or near the opening of the vagina at the same time that an ovum is present in a fallopian tube, pregnancy is possible. It is difficult even for mature women to know exactly when ovulation occurs each cycle, and sperm can live for three to six days in the female reproductive tract. Because there is no reliable way for an adolescent to know when ovulation is going to occur, the risk of pregnancy is always present. Here are some important facts about pregnancy and pregnancy prevention:

- Females can ovulate before their first menstrual period, so a teen can become pregnant before menstruation even starts.

- Sperm normally live for 12 to 48 hours inside the female reproductive tract, but they can live for as long as six days.

- Because the timing of ovulation varies and sperm can live inside the female reproductive tract for several days, fertilization is possible even if sexual intercourse occurs during the female's menstrual period.

- It takes only one sperm and one ovum for pregnancy to occur, and any act of sexual intercourse, even the first, can result in pregnancy.

- Sperm cannot be flushed out of the vagina by urinating; urine leaves the body through the urethra, not the vagina.

GUIDE TO READING

Building Vocabulary

▶ withdrawal
▶ contraception
▶ fertility awareness methods (FAMs)
▶ condom
▶ spermicide
▶ diaphragm
▶ cervical cap
▶ oral contraceptives
▶ contraceptive injection
▶ vasectomy
▶ tubal ligation

Health Concepts

- Analyze the importance of abstinence from sexual activity among teens.
- Recognize abstinence as the only 100 percent effective method in preventing pregnancy and sexually transmitted diseases (STDs), including HIV/AIDS.
- Analyze the effectiveness of contraceptive methods.

Reading Strategy

Predict Scan the headings, subheadings, and photo captions. Write a list of questions you have about the material in this lesson.

Douching is a process used to cleanse the vagina; it is *not* a way to prevent pregnancy:

- Sperm left in or near the opening of the vagina cannot be rinsed out. In fact, the liquid inserted into the vagina during douching actually pushes the sperm upward toward the cervix—the entrance to the uterus.

- Many doctors suggest that females avoid douching. First, douching is unnecessary for cleansing purposes because the vagina cleanses itself. Second, douching can alter the vagina's natural environment and leave a female vulnerable to infection.

- Sperm cannot be flushed out of the vagina by douching; in fact, douching may push sperm farther into the vagina, making fertilization more likely.

- If sexual intercourse occurs while standing up, in a hot tub, or just for a few minutes, pregnancy can occur.

- **Withdrawal**, *the male's removal of the penis from the vagina before ejaculation*, is *not* a reliable method of preventing pregnancy. Some sperm from the ejaculatory duct may be present in the clear fluid released by the Cowper's glands before ejaculation. The male does not know when this pre-ejaculate fluid is being released. Also, if semen is deposited near the outside of the vagina, sperm can travel through vaginal secretions into the vagina. Withdrawing at the height of sexual pleasure also requires a great deal of control at a time when the ability to think clearly and act responsibly is strained.

Contraception

The word **contraception** means *prevention of pregnancy*. As you read about the various forms of contraception, remember that the only 100 percent effective method for preventing pregnancy is abstinence from sexual activity.

Most birth control methods belong to one of the major contraceptive categories:

- Fertility awareness methods (FAM)
- Barrier methods
- Hormonal methods
- Permanent methods

Fertility Awareness Methods (FAMs)

Fertility awareness methods (FAMs) are *methods of contraception that involve determining the fertile days of the female's menstrual cycle and avoiding intercourse during those days*. With typical use, these methods are about 80 percent effective. Because a teen female's menstrual cycle is usually irregular, it is nearly impossible to determine when she ovulates each cycle. Thus, FAMs are a particularly ineffective form of contraception.

The basal body temperature method involves the female taking and recording her temperature every morning before getting out of bed. A basal thermometer is used to identify the slight rise in the female's temperature that occurs at ovulation and continues until she gets her period.

The cervical mucus method requires checking the mucus secretion from the cervix daily and recording changes in its characteristics. Cloudy and sticky for most of the cycle, cervical mucus becomes clear, slippery, and stringy a few days before ovulation.

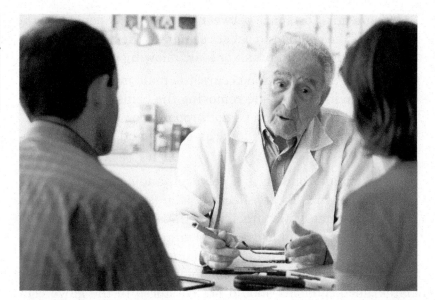

■ **Figure 6.1**
Couples must receive special training from a health care professional to learn how to use FAMs as a form of contraception. *Why is this method not recommended for teens?*

With all FAMs, once the timing of ovulation has been determined, a couple will abstain from intercourse from six or seven days before ovulation until about three days after ovulation. FAMs are entirely dependent on the female having an established, regular menstrual cycle. These methods of contraception provide no protection against STDs.

Barrier Methods

Barrier methods are contraceptive devices that prevent fertilization by keeping sperm from reaching the egg. The sperm are either physically blocked from entering the uterus or spoiled by a chemical before they can reach the egg. The condom, sponge, diaphragm, and cervical cap are all barrier methods that function by blocking the sperm while spermicide acts as a chemical barrier.

The Condom

The male **condom** is *a thin sheath of latex, plastic, or animal tissue that is placed on the erect penis to catch semen. It is a physical barrier to the passage of sperm into the vagina and toward the ovum.* Some condoms are also coated with a **spermicide**, *a chemical that kills sperm.* Condoms can be purchased at drugstores and supermarkets without any prescription or age requirement. For any condom to be an effective contraceptive, it must be used correctly:

- The condom must be unrolled onto the erect penis before there is any contact with the vagina.

Which types of male condoms protect against STDs?

Latex condoms offer the best protection against most STDs, including HIV infection. When used correctly—before there is any sexual contact—they block the exchange of body fluids that may be infected with the pathogens that cause STDs. Polyurethane condoms are also effective, but they are still being studied. Animal-tissue condoms do not offer effective protection against STDs because natural pores in the tissue allow passage of some infectious agents, including HIV. Keep in mind that condoms must be used each and every time sexual intercourse takes place, and instructions must be followed exactly.

- There must be space between the tip of the penis and the end of the condom to collect semen. If there is no space, the condom could break or leak, allowing semen out.

- As soon as ejaculation occurs, the male must hold the condom in place while removing the penis from the vagina. If the condom is not properly removed, once the penis softens, the condom can slip off and release semen into the vagina.

The female condom is a polyurethane pouch that fits inside the vagina. To be effective, it must be inserted before the penis comes in contact with the vagina. Like the male condom, it is available over-the-counter.

Petroleum jelly or other petroleum-based products can dissolve latex and weaken the condom. Since heat also destroys latex, such condoms should not be stored in the glove compartment of a car or carried in a wallet for any length of time. They should be stored in a cool, dry place. Condoms should never be reused; they should be used only once and then discarded.

The Sponge

The sponge is a disc-shaped polyurethane device that contains spermicide. It must be placed in the vagina prior to sexual contact. The sponge must not be removed for at least six hours following sexual activity and should be discarded within 30 hours to prevent toxic shock syndrome. The sponge can be purchased without a prescription.

The Diaphragm and Cervical Cap

The diaphragm, cap, and shield are three barrier devices that can be obtained only with a prescription. A contraceptive **diaphragm** is *a soft latex or silicone cup with a flexible rim that covers the entrance to the cervix*. A **cervical cap** is *a thimble-shaped, soft latex cup that fits snugly over the cervix*. Spermicidal jelly or cream is applied inside both the diaphragm and the cervical cap before insertion.

■ **Figure 6.2**
Diaphragms and cervical caps are barrier methods of contraception because they keep the sperm and ovum apart. Contraceptive implants prevent ovulation.

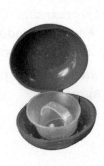
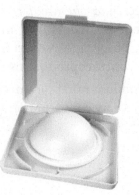

A female needs to have a pelvic examination so that the health care professional can measure her and prescribe the correct diaphragm or cervical cap for her body. A female should be refitted for a diaphragm or a cervical cap if she has delivered a baby, had a miscarriage or an abortion, or either gained or lost more than 15 pounds. The diaphragm or cap must be used correctly every time intercourse takes place:

- **Using the Diaphragm.** The diaphragm must be placed in the vagina prior to sexual activity and left in for at least six hours. If intercourse is repeated, more spermicide must be inserted into the vagina without removing the diaphragm. The diaphragm can be left in the vagina for up to 24 hours.

- **Using the Cervical Cap.** Before inserting the cervical cap, the cup must be one-third full of spermicide. It is important to check that the cervix is completely covered. The cap must stay in place for at least six hours after intercourse, but never for longer than 48 hours.

Spermicide

Contraceptive foams, jellies, creams, and tablets are nonprescription forms of birth control that contain a spermicide. The instructions for each type of spermicide vary, but most are applied by inserting an applicator deep into the vagina, near the cervix. To be effective, the spermicide must be applied between 5 and 90 minutes before intercourse. After intercourse, it is important that the female not bathe or douche; the spermicide must remain in place for six to eight hours to be effective.

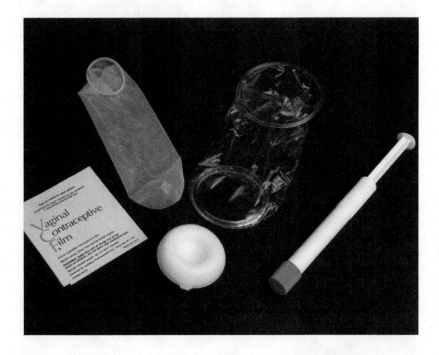

■ **Figure 6.3**
Condoms are one nonprescription method of contraception. Others include contraceptive suppositories and contraceptive foams, jellies, and creams.

Hormonal Methods

Hormonal methods of contraception function by suppressing ovulation and preventing fertilization or implantation. Such methods include oral contraceptives, patches, vaginal contraceptive rings, and contraceptive injections and implants.

The Birth Control Pill

Oral contraceptives, or birth control pills, are *hormone pills that, taken correctly, create changes in the female body that prevent pregnancy*. A health care professional prescribes the birth control pills. The female will be asked to provide a personal and family medical history.

One type of pill is the combined pill, which contains estrogen and progestin. Another type, the mini pill contains only progestin. The pill must be taken every day to be effective. If no pills are ever missed, it is 99.9 percent effective. If a female misses a dose, she should use another method of birth control.

The pill's side effects vary for each individual. For this reason, females should have regular medical checkups and notify a physician if any problem or unusual change occurs. Side effects include nausea, breast tenderness, weight gain, mood swings, and changes in their menstrual cycle. A few develop serious health problems, such as high blood pressure, blood clots, and stroke. Some females, such as those who experience migraine headaches or have diabetes or high blood pressure, or are severely over weight should not take the pill.

■ **Figure 6.4**
To be effective, birth control pills must be taken every day, preferably at the same time of day.

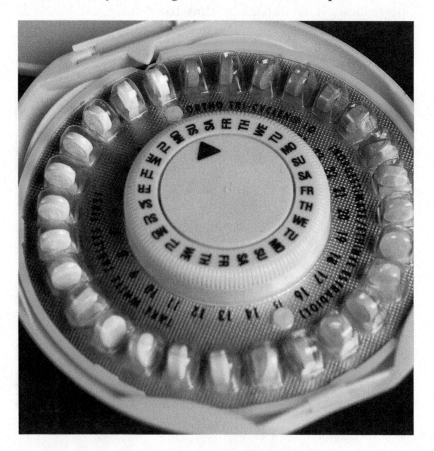

Photo Credit: Christopher Kerrigan/McGraw-Hill Education

The Patch

The patch is a hormonal contraceptive method that works by releasing estrogen and progestin to stop ovulation. It is available through prescription only. The patch can be worn on the lower abdomen, buttocks, or upper body and must be replaced once a week for three weeks each month. Using the patch carries a greater risk for blood clots than using oral contraceptives, and has a 9 percent failure rate.

Vaginal Contraceptive Ring

The vaginal contraceptive ring is another prescribed hormonal contraceptive method that releases progestin and estrogen to stop ovulation. It is a flexible ring that is put into the vagina and left in place for three weeks of every cycle. It is removed during the menstrual period. Another form of birth control should be used if the ring remains out of position for more than three hours. It has a failure rate of 9 percent. Side effects and risks are similar to those of oral contraceptives, but may also include vaginal discharge, swelling, and irritation.

Contraceptive Injection

The **contraceptive injection** is *a birth control procedure in which a female receives an injection once every three months to prevent ovulation.* The shot contains the hormone progestin, which stops ovulation in most women with a 6 percent failure rate. The first injection is generally given during a menstrual cycle or even a few days after a menstrual cycle has started and follow-up injections are required every three months. Risks include breakthrough bleeding, weight gain, breast tenderness, bone loss, and headaches.

Contraceptive Implants

In a contraceptive implant, a thin rod is placed under the skin on the upper arm by a nurse or doctor. The rod releases the hormone progestin, which prevents sperm from fertilizing the egg. This device can remain in the body for up to three years. It is not recommended for women who are overweight or taking medication for tuberculosis, seizures, depression, or HIV/AIDS. It may cause side effects, including ovarian cysts, depression, hair loss, nausea, and changes in the menstrual cycle.

Emergency Contraceptive

A final hormonal method to be used in emergency situations only is the emergency contraceptive method. In the United States, two forms of emergency contraceptives exist. One method consists of taking an emergency contraceptive pill within five days of unprotected sex. The other requires the insertion of a copper IUD within five days of unprotected sexual activity.

Real World CONNECTION

Health Information from Charts and Graphs

You can get useful information from charts and graphs when you know how to read them. The chart below is based on information available from the Food and Drug Administration (FDA). What type of information does this chart give you? Read all the legends and keys to get the maximum information from the chart.

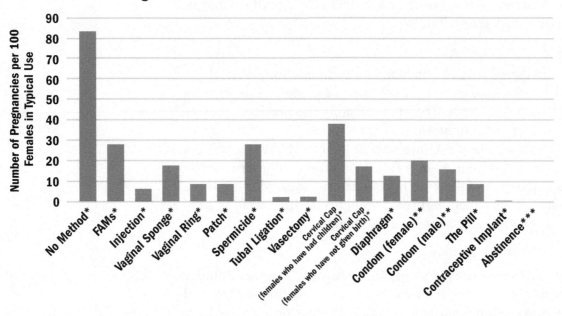

Pregnancies Based on Methods of Birth Control

Source: CDC. Effectiveness of contraceptive methods, www.cdc.gov/reproductive health/Unintended Pregnancy/Contraception.html

Key:
*   No protection against STDs
**   Some protection against STDs
*** Total protection against STDs

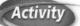 **Activity** Based on the information in the chart, write a summary of the birth control methods covered. In your summary:

- Group methods with similar levels of effectiveness.
- Address the effectiveness of methods that do not fall into any specific group.
- Identify which method is the least effective, which is the most effective, and which offers the most protection against STDs.

Permanent Methods

Permanent contraceptive methods involve a surgical procedure that makes a male or female incapable of reproducing. See **Figure 6.5**. These methods include vasectomy and tubal ligation.

Vasectomy

A **vasectomy** is *a sterilization procedure for males in which each vas deferens is cut and sealed.* It is a method of permanent birth control that works by keeping sperm out of the semen; sperm are still produced but are absorbed by the body rather than mixed into the semen.

Vasectomy does not in any way affect masculinity or the ability to have an erection, to ejaculate, or to experience sexual pleasure. The procedure is 99.9 percent effective. However, the surgery does carry some risks, such as pain, bleeding, and infection. Males who may want to have children someday should not have a vasectomy; surgery to reverse the procedure is costly and has limited success. Vasectomy does not protect the male or the female against STDs.

■ **Figure 6.5**
Sterilization Methods

In a vasectomy, each vas deferens is cut and sealed off. During a tubal ligation, the fallopian tubes are cut and tied or clamped off to prevent sperm from reaching the ova.

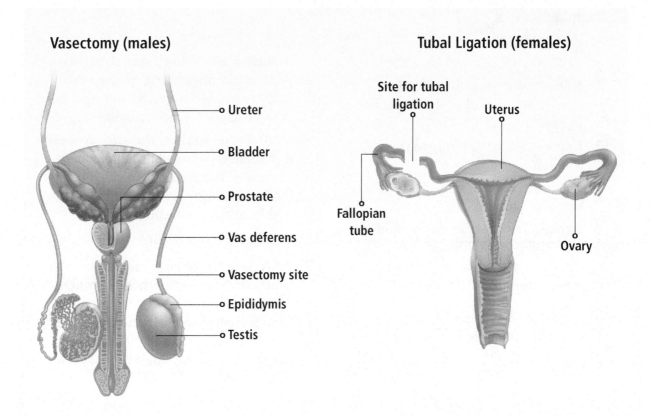

Vasectomy (males)

- Ureter
- Bladder
- Prostate
- Vas deferens
- Vasectomy site
- Epididymis
- Testis

Tubal Ligation (females)

- Site for tubal ligation
- Uterus
- Fallopian tube
- Ovary

Tubal Ligation

Tubal ligation is *a sterilization procedure for females in which the fallopian tubes are cut and tied or clamped to prevent sperm from reaching the ova.* An ovum is still released each month, but it cannot be fertilized and dissolves inside the body. Tubal ligation is a more involved procedure than vasectomy and requires a hospital stay. Complications following surgery may include cramps, heavier periods, breakthrough bleeding, and pelvic pain. Tubal ligation is 99.5 percent effective and is considered permanent. Surgery to reverse the procedure has met with limited success in restoring fertility. As with vasectomy, this method of birth control offers no protection against STDs, including HIV/AIDS.

Abstinence

Abstinence from sexual activity is the only 100 percent effective method for preventing pregnancy and STDs. By making a decision to abstain from sexual activity, you demonstrate maturity and a positive self-concept, and you preserve your chances of fulfilling your goals for the future.

LESSON 1 ASSESSMENT

After You Read
Reviewing Facts and Vocabulary

1. Name two hormonal methods of contraception and explain how each works.

2. Explain the proper way to use a male condom.

3. List four possible side effects of the birth control pill.

4. Explain how barrier methods of contraception work. Identify one method that is designed for males and one that is designed for females.

Thinking Critically

5. Analyze. Using a scale of 1 to 5 (with 1 being the most effective), analyze the effectiveness and ineffectiveness of each of the following contraceptive methods in preventing pregnancy: diaphragm, birth control pill, spermicide, abstinence, male condom.

6. Synthesize. Analyze the effectiveness and ineffectiveness of the following contraceptive methods in preventing STDs: diaphragm, birth control pill, FAMs, abstinence, condom.

Applying Health Skills

7. Advocacy. Create a poster that compares various methods of contraception and shows why abstinence from sexual activity is the only birth control method that is 100 percent effective in preventing pregnancy and STDs, including HIV/AIDS.

Concerns About Sexuality

Quick Write

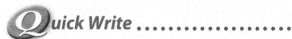

Write a list of questions you have about sexuality. After reading the lesson, review your list and consider talking to a trusted adult about any remaining questions or concerns.

Your sexuality is part of your personality, and will begin developing during your teen years. Developing feelings of attraction is a normal response to the changes you are experiencing. Many of these new feelings, however, can be difficult to talk about. If you have questions, try talking to a trusted adult. Reluctance to learn the facts about sexuality can have a significant impact on your health.

Sexual Orientation

Sexual orientation is the recognition of a gender preference with regard to sexual attraction. What causes sexual orientation? No single reason exists as to why people are attracted to other people. According to the American Psychological Association, sexual orientation is the result of an interaction of cognitive, environmental, and biological factors.

People use many different labels to describe their sexual orientation and gender identity. A few of the most common are:

- **Homosexual** describes *someone who is sexually attracted to people of the same gender*.
- **Bisexual** describes *an individual who is sexually attracted to people of both genders*.
- Heterosexual describes an individual who is attracted to people of the opposite sex.
- **Transgender** describes *an individual whose gender identity differs from others of their gender*. They can be heterosexual, homosexual, or bisexual. A transgender person may choose to live as his or her opposite gender.

GUIDE TO READING

Building Vocabulary
- homosexual
- bisexual
- transgender
- intersexual
- LGBTQ
- stereotype
- masturbation
- abortion

Health Concepts
- Explain why some people masturbate.
- Describe myths regarding sexual orientation.
- Distinguish between spontaneous and induced abortion.

Reading Strategy
Explain Write down the Building Vocabulary terms and include a definition for each in your own words. After reading the lesson, compare your definitions to those in the text.

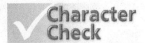

Respect When you show empathy and tolerance for people who are different from you, you are demonstrating respect.
Imagine you overhear your nine-year-old brother telling a friend that someone is homosexual. You are concerned that your brother is stereotyping. Write what you would say to him.

- **Intersexual** describes *an individual who was born with both male and female characteristics.*
- Questioning describes an individual who questions their own identity and orientation.
- **LGBTQ** is a common acronym meaning *lesbian, gay, bisexual, transgender, or questioning.*

The topic of sexuality is one that causes a great deal of controversy, and has resulted in the formation of many myths. Some believe that a person is homosexual if he or she has a close friendship with a member of the same gender. Another is that if a person has not had a sexual relationship by a certain age, he or she is homosexual. Some people believe that someone who is attracted to members of the same gender can change and become heterosexual. Finally, some people believe that having certain mannerisms and behaviors is an indication of person's sexual orientation. All of these myths are untrue. In fact, the final myth is also a **stereotype**, or *an idea or image held about a group of people that represents a prejudiced attitude, oversimplified opinion, or uninformed judgment.*

Coming Out

Coming out refers to identifying oneself with a certain sexual orientation, and telling others. A person who comes out has made the difficult decision to let others know that he or she views himself or herself as a LGBTQ person. The person coming out is the only person who can decide when to come out, who to tell, and how the message should be shared.

The person coming out should consider carefully who he or she will tell. Some things to thing about before coming out include:

- What are the reasons for coming out? A good reason is to develop a more honest relationship with another person. Coming out to hurt someone when angry can have negative consequences. Wait until the anger passes to come out.
- Is it possible that the person will become physically harmful? Only come out if you feel that the person will be accepting and supportive.
- Will the other person honor the privacy of the person coming out? Is there any chance that the person will use teasing or tell others without permission? If so, avoid coming out to this person.

■ **Figure 6.6**
Throughout the life cycle, it is normal and healthy to have close friendships with peers of the same gender. Such friendships have no bearing on sexual orientation.

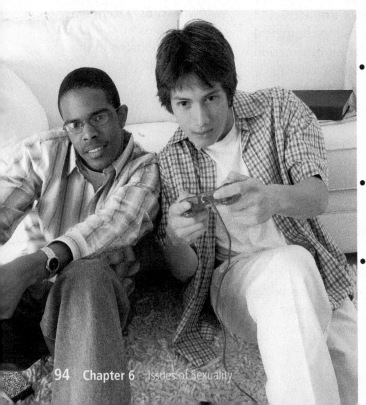

Finally, when a person comes out, he or she should understand that the person hearing the announcement may be surprised. That person may say things that feel hurtful because of that surprise. Give the person time to absorb the information. In some cases, sharing information on sexual orientation may change friendship. Some friendships may end.

If a friend tells you that he or she is LGBTQ, keep in mind that he or she has had these feelings for quite a while. Some LGBTQ people report feelings of attraction to the same gender or both genders beginning at a young age. Others may not begin recognizing these feelings until later in life. Others may feel that they were born with the incorrect set of genitals, and should be the other gender. A friend will continue to show respect for the person who has come out, and to allow him or her to choose when and with whom to share the information.

Finally, teens who are struggling with coming out have a resource. The Trevor Project operates a free, 24-hour, 7-day-a-week hotline (1-866-488-7386) for LGBTQ youth. Staff who take calls are trained to help LGBTQ teens. All calls are confidential meaning that the information shared between the teen and a counselor will not be shared with others.

Dating

Dating is a way to get to know other people better. For a LGBTQ teen, though, dating can be very difficult. LGBTQ teens who are open about their orientation may have difficulty finding other teens in their school to date. A community with a youth organization for LGBTQ teens may be a place to connect with other teens.

Declining a date

Asking a person out on a date can be a very difficult experience. A person who is known for a long time may be a good person to ask on a date, but if that person wants to be only friends, he or she may decline the date. For LGBTQ teens, dating can be even more difficult. Some teens may feel threatened by the sexual orientation of an LGBTQ teen. Other may feel that they are LGBTQ as well, but are not ready to come out. In these instances, your goal should be to decline the date, but maintain the friendship. Be respectful. Tell the other person no, but that you want to remain friends. If you feel comfortable, tell the person why you are saying no.

Masturbation

Masturbation means *touching one's own genitals for sexual pleasure.* Some people believe that masturbation is a natural part of growth and development, while others believe it is wrong and unhealthy. Masturbation is a personal issue and a private activity. People masturbate to relieve sexual tension. It is natural, unless the behavior becomes obsessive, or extremely habitual.

Pregnancy Termination

Another topic related to sexuality is pregnancy termination, or abortion, any termination of a pregnancy. Pregnancies end prematurely for many reason. When a pregnancy ends spontaneously from natural causes, it is called a spontaneous abortion, or a miscarriage. Miscarriages most commonly occur in the first trimester of pregnancy, and can affect as many as 25 percent of all pregnancies. In some cases, a female may not even be aware that she is pregnant.

A medical terminated pregnancy, also called an induced abortion, purposely ends a pregnancy. An induced abortion is a medical procedure and must be performed by qualified professionals in a medical setting. The issue of induced abortion is highly controversial and should never be considered a method of birth control.

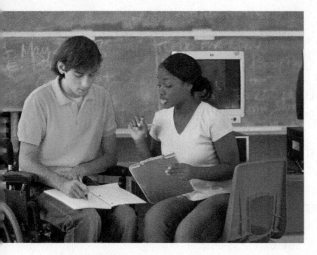

■ Figure 6.7
Teens in schools across the nation are finding ways to promote tolerance and respect.

Photo Credit: Tim Fuller Photography

LESSON 2 ASSESSMENT

After You Read
Reviewing Facts and Vocabulary

1. Define the terms *homosexual*, *bisexual*, and *heterosexual*.

2. What is a *stereotype*?

3. What are some myths about sexual orientation? Explain why they are unfounded.

Thinking Critically

4. **Analyze.** Why can stereotypes harm people?

5. **Synthesize.** Why do you think people have such strong viewpoints about induced abortion?

Applying Health Skills

6. **Communication Skills.** Write a paragraph explaining what you would say to a friend who tells you that she is concerned about her sexual orientation because she has not started dating yet.

Sexual Abuse and Violence

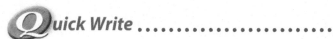 *uick Write* ....

> *Write a public service announcement providing teens with information about what to do if they are the victim of sexual abuse or violence.*

When an act of sexual contact is forced on a person, it is an act of violence. The force that is used against the victim may be physical or emotional.

Sexual Abuse and Incest

Sexual abuse is *any sexual contact that is physically or emotionally forced on a person against his or her will*. Sexual abuse is always illegal, it is always a crime, and it is never the victim's fault. It can affect people of all social, economic, and ethnic groups. Males and females of any age may be victims of sexual abuse. Many times, the victim knows the abuser.

If the sexual abuser is related to the victim, the abuse is called **incest**—*sexual contact between family members who cannot marry by law*. Incest can involve parents or stepparents, aunts, uncles, brothers, sisters, or any other relative. If the sexual abuser is a trusted adult, the pressure used against a young victim is commonly persuasive or emotional rather than physical. The adult may discourage the victim from telling anyone about the abuse by using statements such as:

- "This will be our special secret."
- "Telling will break up the family."
- "I'll go to jail and it will be your fault."
- "No one will believe you, and I'll say you're lying."
- "Your parents will be very mad at/disappointed in you."

These types of statements are very persuasive because they can provoke guilt and anxiety in young people. Some victims may believe they caused the abuse or that they were at fault because they did not resist. Remember that, without exception, sexual abuse is the fault of the abuser, not the victim.

GUIDE TO READING

Building Vocabulary
- ▶ sexual abuse
- ▶ incest
- ▶ rape
- ▶ acquaintance rape
- ▶ date rape

Health Concepts
- Analyze issues surrounding sexual abuse and incest.
- Describe situations that can lead to acquaintance rape and date rape.
- Analyze the importance of healthy strategies that prevent physical, sexual, and emotional abuse.

Reading Strategy
Predict Scan the headings, subheadings, and photo captions. Write a list of questions you have about the material in this lesson.

What to Do About Sexual Abuse

The first and most important step a victim of sexual abuse can take is to tell someone about the abuse. This is particularly difficult to do if the abuser is a family member, a friend of the family, or a leader within the community. People might not believe the victim because they can't imagine that the accused person could be a sexual abuser. Both the victim and the abuser need professional help and counseling.

Rape

Rape, or *any form of sexual intercourse that takes place against a person's will*, is illegal. As with other types of sexual abuse, rape is an act of violence. Victims of rape can be males or females of any age. In the United States, more than 84,000 forcible rapes were reported in 2012.

Health Skills Activity

Decision Making

Dealing with an Unsafe Dating Situation

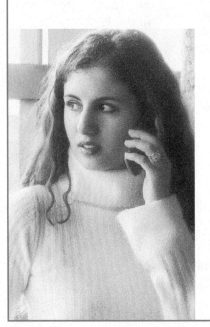

Carrie was home baby sitting her little sister one Saturday night when the phone rang.

"Carrie? Thank goodness you're home."

"Betsy, what's wrong? Where are you?"

"I'm in Will's bathroom," Betsy whispered. "I'm so scared!"

"What's going on?"

"Will's parents are out for the night. We started kissing, but then Will got angry with me when I didn't want to go any farther than that. What should I do, Carrie? Will's waiting for me to come back. I need your help."

What Would You Do?
Put yourself in Carrie's shoes. Apply the six steps of the decision-making process to help Carrie decide how to help her friend.
1. State the situation.
2. List the options.
3. Weigh the possible outcomes.
4. Consider values.
5. Make a decision and act on it.
6. Evaluate the decision.

Many rapes of female teens are either **acquaintance rape**, *rape by someone the victim knows,* or **date rape**, *rape by someone the victim is dating.* A victim of date or acquaintance rape may think it wasn't rape because she knows the male, or she may feel responsible for a rape because she didn't resist soon enough or firmly enough. Whenever any sexual act is forced on a person against his or her will, it is rape, and rape is never the victim's fault.

The best ways to reduce the occurrence of rape is for all victims to report it. Although the reporting procedure can be difficult, embarrassing, or upsetting, an unreported rape leaves the rapist uncaught, unpunished, and free to rape again.

Reduce Your Risk of Rape

Follow these guidelines to reduce your risk of rape:

- Do not go places alone; stay with a group.
- If you do go somewhere alone, tell someone your plans.
- Walk briskly, be aware of your surroundings, and look alert.
- Stay in well-lit areas where other people are present.
- Have your keys out and ready as you approach your home or car.
- Lock all doors and keep windows up when driving; check inside and under a parked car before getting in.
- Keep windows and doors locked at home; never open your door to strangers.
- If you have car trouble, stay inside your locked car. If someone offers to help, remain in your car and ask the person to call for assistance.
- Keep a cell phone in your purse or car.
- If you are being followed, go to a public place. Run, scream, and make as much noise as you can.

Protecting Yourself Against Date Rape

Use these tips to protect yourself against date rape:

- Do not go on blind dates unless you are with a group. Know the person you are going out with.
- Go on group dates the first few times you're out with a new person.
- Do not go to isolated places on a date.
- Tell someone at home where you will be and when you plan to return.
- Take money with you, including change, so that you can make a phone call or take a taxi home if a situation becomes unsafe. If you have a cell phone, bring it.
- Do not use drugs or alcohol. If your date is using these substances, leave immediately.

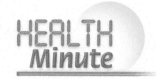

Avoid Becoming a Victim of Date Rape Drugs

The term *date rape drugs* is used to describe the drugs Rohypnol, GHB, and ketamine, which rapists sometimes give to unknowing victims, usually by dissolving the drug in a drink. These drugs cause blackouts and memory loss, leaving a victim helpless, unaware of what is happening, and unable to recall what happened.

To protect yourself against date rape drugs:

- Never accept any kind of drink from someone you don't know well and trust completely.
- Never accept a drink you have not seen poured or made.
- Do not leave your drink unattended.
- Do not accept a drink from a large public beverage container, such as a punch bowl.
- If you feel ill, ask for help immediately and publicly.

What to Do If You or Someone You Know Is Raped

Being raped is a terrifying experience. If you or someone you know has been raped, do the following:

- Tell a parent, close friend, or someone else you trust; ask for emotional support.

- Notify the police immediately. Ask for a sex crimes officer of the same gender as you are.

- Do not take a shower, change clothes, or douche. These actions can remove evidence that the police will need.

- Get a physical examination as soon as possible. Most rape victims have injuries that need medical attention. A hospital emergency room is equipped to handle rape cases and can collect evidence to help identify the rapist.

- Find a counselor, therapist, or support group to help work through the emotional trauma of rape. It is normal for a rape victim to have a wide range of feelings. Many communities have a rape crisis center with counselors who are specially trained for this purpose.

LESSON 3 ASSESSMENT

After You Read
Reviewing Facts and Vocabulary

1. Define the term *sexual abuse*.

2. Why might a victim of sexual abuse or incest remain silent about the abuse?

3. What is the first and most important step a victim of sexual abuse can take?

4. List three things you can do to protect yourself against date rape.

5. Why shouldn't a victim of rape take a shower or change clothes afterward?

Thinking Critically

6. **Analyze.** What is the difference between sexual abuse and incest?

7. **Synthesize.** List five situations a person could be in that might put him or her at risk of being a victim of rape. Suggest ways this person can make better decisions to protect himself or herself.

Applying Health Skills

8. **Practicing Healthful Behaviors.** Analyze the importance of healthy strategies to prevent physical, sexual, and emotional abuse, including date rape. Create a pamphlet that features tips for teens on how to protect themselves against rape. Use appealing design elements and colors to illustrate your pamphlet. Distribute the pamphlets throughout your school.

Reviewing Facts and Vocabulary

1. Why is douching not an effective method of contraception?

2. What is *withdrawal*? Is it an effective method of preventing pregnancy?

3. Name two forms of permanent contraception.

4. List two fertility awareness methods of contraception.

5. Name three prescription forms of birth control.

6. What are *oral contraceptives*?

7. How long does a contraceptive implant provide protection from pregnancy?

8. What is the term for a pregnancy that ends spontaneously?

9. What is *rape*?

10. Explain the difference between *acquaintance rape* and *date rape*.

Writing Critically

11. Synthesize. Write a summary describing what you would do if you received conflicting information about contraception. Where would you go to find the correct information?

12. Compare. Write a summary comparing vasectomy and tubal ligation in terms of the actual procedure and effectiveness.

13. Synthesize. Using facts from this chapter, write an analysis of the importance of abstinence from sexual activity as the preferred choice of behavior for an unmarried person of school age.

14. Analyze. Write a report explaining why you think some people believe false information about sexual issues, such as homosexuality or bisexuality.

15. Evaluate. Write a paragraph describing how a child who has been sexually abused might be helped by a counselor who specializes in such cases.

Applying Health Skills

16. Accessing Information. Create a directory of all the resources available in your community to help people with contraception, STDs, sexual abuse, and rape.

17. Analyzing Influences. How might movies that feature people making unsafe decisions about sexual activity negatively affect a teen audience?

Activity Beyond the Classroom

Parent Involvement
Discuss safety strategies. With a parent or guardian, discuss ways that teens can reduce the risk of date or acquaintance rape.

School and Community
Help for victims. Do research at the library and talk to a counselor about treatment of victims of rape and incest. Write a report about the treatment process and add suggestions that you feel might help victims. Suggest ways that present treatment methods might be improved.

CHAPTER 7

Sexually Transmitted Diseases

Photo Credit Jeremie Westbrook/Blend Images/Getty Images

Activating Prior Knowledge

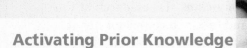 List sources of information teens can access on STDs or STIs. In addition to medical professionals and pamphlets, what other sources could teens use to find accurate information?

Common Sexually Transmitted Diseases

GUIDE TO READING

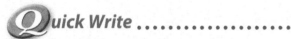uick Write ....

Write down the questions you have about STDs. If your questions are not answered after reading the lesson, talk to a trusted adult about any additional concerns related to this topic.

Great strides have been made in controlling the spread of many communicable diseases, but the incidence of sexually transmitted diseases continues to rise. **Sexually transmitted diseases** (STDs), more commonly known as sexually transmitted infections (STIs), are *infections that spread from person to person through sexual contact*. There are more than 25 known STDs, many of which are difficult to track because people who have them may not exhibit symptoms. Other cases are not reported because people do not seek treatment due to shame, fear, or ignorance.

STDs: Widespread Among Teens

An estimated 20 million people contract one or more STDs in the United States each year. About half of these new cases involve those between the ages of 13 and 24. Currently in the United States, more than 110 million people have an STD. Why do these epidemics persist and grow? One reason is that many STDs have no symptoms. Other STDs have a lengthy delay between infection and the appearance of symptoms, and still others have symptoms that go away while the disease continues to damage the body. Many people also remain uneducated about STDs or believe that they are somehow immune.

Building Vocabulary

- sexually transmitted diseases (STDs)
- human papillomavirus (HPV)
- genital warts
- chlamydia
- pelvic inflammatory disease (PID)
- gonorrhea
- genital herpes

Health Concepts

- Describe the relationship between high-risk behaviors and the risk of contracting an STD.
- Discuss abstinence from sexual activity as the only method that is 100 percent effective in preventing STDs.
- Develop and analyze strategies to prevent the spread of STDs.

Reading Strategy

Problems and Solutions
Write a brief summary describing some of the behaviors you think can expose someone to an STD or STI. Add a list of tips to prevent the transmission of these diseases and infections.

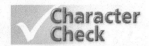

Responsibility Saying no to sexual activity is an important way to take responsibility for your health.

Make a list of reasons to practice abstinence. For example, "I value my health." Think about how these can be used as part of your refusal strategies if you are pressured to engage in sexual activity.

Sexually active teens have a high risk for contracting STDs because teens who are sexually active are likely to engage in one or more of the following behaviors:

- Engaging in any form of unprotected intercourse—including oral, anal, or vaginal sexual contact—without using any barrier protection method such as condoms
- Using alcohol and other drugs, which can change people's behavior and lower their inhibitions
- Being sexually active with multiple partners
- Engaging in any sexual relationship
- Choosing partners who have a history of intravenous drug use
- Choosing a partner who seems to be low risk but is not

Abstinence Can Prevent STDs

Some teens may think that only people who engage in sexual intercourse get STDs. The truth is that anyone who has sexual contact with an infected person is at risk. Because a person who has an STD does not always show symptoms, sexual activity of any kind with any person is risky. The good news is that STDs can be prevented. Choosing to practice abstinence is a healthy, responsible, and mature decision for teens. Here are some guidelines that teens can follow to avoid risky situations:

- Set limits and communicate them to your date before you go out.
- Stay in public places when you go on dates.
- Use refusal strategies if you are pressured to engage in sexual activity.
- Never use alcohol or illegal drugs.
- Choose friends and dates who practice abstinence.
- Protect your food and beverages to avoid the risk of date rape drugs.
- Use latex condoms to provide the best protection against most STDs.

Common STDs in the United States

In this lesson, you will learn important facts about some of the most common STDs—human papillomavirus, chlamydia, gonorrhea, and genital herpes. The most important fact to remember is: the primary way these STDs are spread is through any form of sexual intercourse, including vaginal, oral, or anal sex.

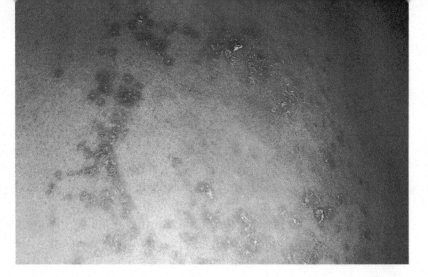

■ Figure 7.1
Barrier protection methods such as condoms are not effective in preventing HPV. The virus can be transmitted without the presence of genital warts.

Human Papillomavirus

Human papillomavirus (HPV) is *a virus that causes genital warts and warts on other parts of the body.* While chlamydia is the most commonly *reported* STD in the United States, health experts believe that genital HPV infection is the most commonly *contracted* of all STDs. Though many cases go unnoticed and unreported, it is believed that about 14 million people contract HPV each year in the United States.

Like many STDs, HPV infection often does not have symptoms. The most easily recognized symptom is **genital warts** (also called venereal warts), which are *soft, moist, pink or red swellings that appear on the genitals and are caused by the human papillomavirus.* In females, the warts are found on the vulva, in the vagina, on the cervix, or around the anus. In males, genital warts are found on the penis, on the scrotum, or around the anus. Genital warts are found only rarely in the mouth or throat.

There are more than 100 types of HPV, most of which are harmless and cause benign conditions such as skin warts on other parts of the body. Certain types of genital HPV infection are linked to cervical cancer, including some that are also associated with cancers of the vulva, anus, and penis. A vaccine that can prevent HPV is now available and is recommended for pre-teens from age 11 or 12. Individuals up to age 26 are encouraged to be vaccinated to prevent HPV. The vaccine may reduce the number of cases of cervical cancer caused by certain types of HPV.

HPV is most commonly diagnosed through an examination of genital warts. Doctors sometimes use an acidic solution to make warts more visible. Genital warts may disappear by themselves, or they can be removed by laser or by being frozen, burned, or cut off. An antiviral drug can also be injected directly into larger warts, and other topical treatments may be used. Removal of the warts does not eliminate the virus, however. The warts can recur.

Chlamydia

Chlamydia is *an STD that is caused by the bacterium* Chlamydia trachomatis. The highest incidence of chlamydia in the United States is among teens and young adults. About 1.5 million people in the U.S are diagnosed with chlamydia each year. However, health officials estimate that the actual number is almost 3 million. This discrepancy is a result of the fact that chlamydia may has no symptoms in many people.

During the early stages of infection, females can develop an abnormal vaginal discharge or a burning sensation when urinating. Males with symptoms may have a discharge from the penis and a burning sensation when urinating. If symptoms of early infection do occur, they usually appear within one to three weeks of sexual contact with an infected person. Untreated infections may spread to other reproductive organs in both males and females, often without symptoms until permanent damage has occurred. A pregnant female can spread chlamydia to her baby during delivery, causing eye infections and sometimes pneumonia.

Diagnosis of chlamydia is made by collecting a specimen from the infected site and testing for bacteria. A more recent test involves checking a urine sample for bacteria. If chlamydia is diagnosed, antibiotics can easily cure the infection.

About 40 percent of females with untreated chlamydia will develop **pelvic inflammatory disease** (PID), *a painful infection of the uterus, fallopian tubes, and/or ovaries*. Permanent damage to these structures can result, along with severe pelvic pain, infertility, and an increased likelihood of ectopic pregnancy. An active chlamydia infection also makes a female three to five times more likely to become infected with HIV if she is exposed to the virus.

Gonorrhea

Gonorrhea is *an STD caused by bacteria that live in warm, moist areas of the body, such as mucous membranes*. With more than 820,000 new cases reported each year in the United States, gonorrhea is an extremely common infectious disease. The bacterium *Neisseria gonorrhoeae* causes gonorrhea. This organism can thrive in mucous membranes of the cervix, uterus, and fallopian tubes in females, and in the urethra, mouth, throat, and anus of both females and males.

Teens and young adults have the highest incidence of gonorrhea. Among females, 15- to 19-year-olds have the highest reported rate; among males, the highest rate is among 20- to 24-year-olds.

Most males do show some symptoms of the disease when they are infected. These usually appear two to ten days after infection. Symptoms of genital infection include a burning sensation when urinating, a white, yellow, or green discharge from the penis, and sometimes painful or swollen testicles.

In females, the disease may go unnoticed because females often show no symptoms. Early symptoms in females are often so mild they are mistaken for another type of infection. Symptomatic females have a burning sensation when urinating and a yellow vaginal discharge that is sometimes tinged with blood. In a rectal infection, symptoms in both males and females may include anal discharge, itching, soreness, and bleeding, as well as painful bowel movements. Throat infection causes few symptoms.

Untreated gonorrhea in females can lead to PID. In males, gonorrhea can cause epididymitis, an inflammation of the testicles that can cause sterility. Gonorrhea can also affect the prostate gland and cause scarring inside the urethra. In both sexes, gonorrhea can spread to the blood or joints, at which point the disease becomes life threatening.

Gonorrhea is treated with antibiotics. Chlamydia infection is often present in people with gonorrhea, so antibiotics to treat both conditions are usually given at the same time. People with gonorrhea are more likely to contract HIV if exposed; those with both HIV infection and gonorrhea are also more likely to spread HIV.

Genital Herpes

Genital herpes is *an STD caused by the herpes simplex virus. Herpes simplex 1 usually causes cold sores in or near the mouth.* According to the CDC, almost 20 percent of all people in the United States currently have the disease. Almost 800,000 new cases are reported each year.

A person infected with genital herpes frequently has no symptoms. If symptoms do occur, it is usually within two to five days of exposure but may take up to 30 days. Symptoms consist of an outbreak of blisters on or around the genitals or rectum. Some people may also have a fever and swollen glands. After the blisters break, painful lesions remain that take two to four weeks to heal. Within a few weeks or months, another outbreak may occur, but it is usually less severe than the first. A person may have four or five such episodes in the first year but fewer as the years go by.

The virus is spread from open sores during sexual contact, but it also can be transmitted when lesions are not present. One reason so many people have herpes simplex virus type 2 (HSV-2) is that once a person has been infected, he or she will always have the disease and can spread it to other people.

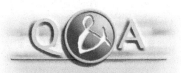

What are a sexually active person's chances of contracting an STD?

Sexually active individuals are at high risk of contracting an STD. Three million teens contract an STD each year. One out of every four Americans will contract an STD at some point in their lifetime. About 75 percent of sexually active people have been infected with HPV. More than 20 percent have genital herpes. In one single act of unprotected sex with an infected person, a female teen has a 30 percent chance of getting genital herpes and a 50 percent chance of getting gonorrhea.

Certain antiviral medications can reduce the duration and severity of episodes, but the virus itself remains forever in the person's system. Consistent and correct use of condoms can help protect against infections. However, condoms may not completely cover the sores and the virus can still spread.

HSV-2 can be fatal to newborns if contracted from the mother during delivery. Pregnant females who have an active genital herpes infection usually have a cesarean delivery to protect the baby.

Herpes simplex virus type 1 (HSV-1) is also common in the United States but is not considered an STD. HSV-1 causes cold sores, which are blisters on the mouth and lips of infected people. The virus can be spread by saliva to another person, or through kissing and touching when lesions are present. An HSV-1 infection can occur on the genitals following oral-genital contact with a person who has a cold sore.

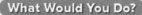

Health Skills Activity

Communication

Helping a Friend Solve a Problem

Jenna and Madison grew up next door to each other and have always been good friends. Madison takes Jenna aside one day after school.

"I'm scared, Jen. You've got to help me."

Jenna winces as Madison explains what's wrong.

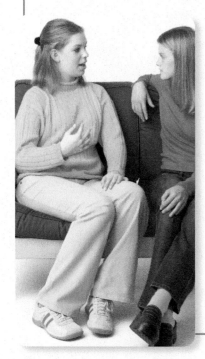

"I've got these blisters on my...you know...down there. They're turning into really painful sores."

Jenna shakes her head in sympathy. Madison adds, "I don't even know how I got whatever this is—Andre and I have fooled around a little, but we've never done that much. He promised me he'd never done anything with anyone else!"

"Oh, Madison," Jenna says.

"Don't judge me, Jen. Just tell me what I'm supposed to do."

Jenna wonders what she should say to Madison.

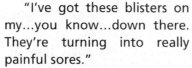

What Would You Do?

Write a dialogue showing how Jenna can use good communication to advise Madison.

1. Use "I" statements to tell how you feel.
2. Keep your tone respectful.
3. Provide a clear, organized message that states the problem.
4. Listen to the other person's side without interrupting.

Photo Credit: Ken Karp/McGraw-Hill Education

Oral-genital contact with a person who has HSV-2 can also cause HSV-2 infection on the mouth. Anyone who is having an active episode of HSV-1 or HSV-2 should avoid touching the lesions. Careful personal hygiene, including hand washing, helps prevent the spread of the herpes virus to other people and other areas of one's own body.

Remember that abstinence is the only 100 percent effective method to avoid contracting STDs. You can protect yourself from the risks of STDs by practicing abstinence from sexual activity before marriage and by using refusal skills to avoid situations in which you may be at risk. Choosing friends who support your decision to remain abstinent will help you in your commitment.

LESSON 1 ASSESSMENT

After You Read
Reviewing Facts and Vocabulary

1. Define *sexually transmitted diseases*. Explain why they are difficult to track.

2. Describe the relationship between high-risk behaviors and the risk for contracting STDs.

3. What is *human papillomavirus* and how common is it?

4. Name three things you can do to reduce your risk of contracting an STD.

5. Name some of the results of untreated gonorrhea.

Thinking Critically

6. Synthesize. You and a friend have agreed to help each other remain abstinent. Your friend has just told you that she has accepted a date with a boy who has a reputation for being sexually active. What would you tell your friend about developing strategies to prevent the spread of STDs?

7. Compare. How are the early symptoms for chlamydia and gonorrhea similar?

Applying Health Skills

8. Practicing Healthful Behaviors. Communicate the importance of practicing abstinence from sexual activity. Make a pamphlet with guidelines teens can follow to avoid risky situations and behaviors that may compromise their decision to practice abstinence.

GUIDE TO READING

Building Vocabulary

▶ hepatitis B (HBV)
▶ syphilis
▶ vaginitis
▶ trichomoniasis
▶ bacterial vaginosis (BV)
▶ pubic lice
▶ scabies

Health Concepts

• Develop and analyze strategies to prevent spreading STDs.
• Identify, describe, and assess community health services available for prevention and treatment of STDs.
• Analyze the importance of abstinence in the prevention of STDs.

Reading Strategy

Problems and Solutions
Write a brief summary describing some of the behaviors that you think can expose someone to an STD. Add a list of tips to prevent the transmission of these STDs.

■ **Figure 7.2**
Hepatitis B is transmitted through contact with the blood of someone who is infected, and can be spread through needles used for body piercing or tattoos.

Other Sexually Transmitted Diseases

*Q*uick Write ....

List two or more effects of STDs. Write two refusal skills you can use to avoid contracting an STD.

Hepatitis B

Hepatitis B (HBV) is *a viral STD that attacks the liver and can cause extreme illness and death.* HBV is transmitted when blood or other body fluids from an infected person enter the body of a person who is not immune to the disease. The virus can be spread through sexual activity or the use of unclean needles. Sharing needles for drug use or having body piercings and tattoos are high-risk behaviors. An infected mother can also pass the virus to her baby during delivery.

An estimated 2,000 die from infections or illness caused by HBV. About 422,000 people now have a chronic sexually acquired HBV infection.

When HBV symptoms occur, they include jaundice, fatigue, abdominal pain, nausea and vomiting, joint pain, and loss of appetite.

A vaccine against HBV has been available since 1982 and is routinely given to children from birth to age 18. Health care and public safety workers, and anyone else exposed to blood or other body fluids, should also be vaccinated against HBV.

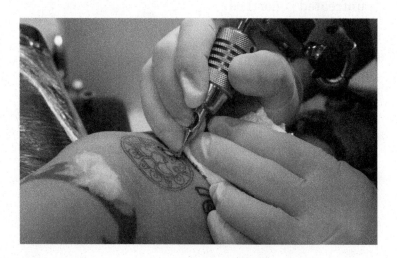

Hepatitis C

According to the CDC, more than 3 million Americans have been infected with the hepatitis C virus. About 16,000 new cases are reported each year. This disease can lead to chronic liver disease, liver cancer, and liver failure. Chronic hepatitis C is often asymptomatic, and the disease progresses slowly. Infected individuals may not realize they have the disease until damage is detected during a routine physical examination. Hepatitis C is transmitted through sexual contact and other direct contact with contaminated blood, such as contaminated needles used in injected drugs. A therapy combining specific drugs can reduce the effects of hepatitis C, but there is no 100 percent cure.

Syphilis

Syphilis is *an STD caused by the bacterium* Treponema pallidum; *it progresses in stages.* Left untreated, syphilis causes severe, sometimes fatal damage to internal organs. In the U.S, about 50,000 new cases of syphilis are reported each year.

Syphilis is spread by direct contact with a chancre, a painless sore that appears early in the disease, or by contact with the infectious rash that appears later. Syphilis is transmitted primarily through sexual activity, including vaginal, oral, and anal sex. Pregnant females who have untreated syphilis can pass the disease to the fetus during pregnancy, which can cause stillbirth or the death of the infant shortly after birth. Infected infants who receive no treatment may have developmental delays, have seizures, or die from the disease.

■ **Figure 7.3**
In the United States today, three doses of hepatitis B vaccine are routinely administered to infants. Children and adolescents who were not immunized as infants receive the vaccine during later visits to their pediatrician.

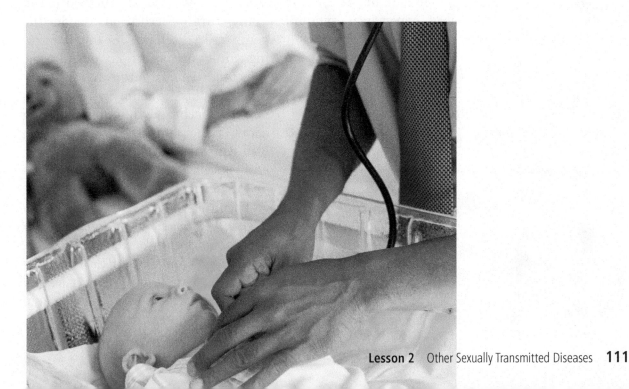

Untreated syphilis progresses through three stages:

Primary Stage. Within 10 to 90 days of infection, a small, firm, round sore called a chancre appears at the spot where the bacterium entered the body. The sore is painless and lasts for three to six weeks, after which it disappears, even without treatment.

Secondary Stage. An infectious rash of rough, red or reddish-brown spots appears on the palms of the hands and the soles of the feet. Flu-like symptoms, hair loss, and weight loss can also be present. The rash disappears without treatment.

Late Syphilis. During a latent period usually lasting several years, external signs of the disease disappear. The organism remains in the body, however, damaging organs such as the brain, nerves, eyes, heart, blood vessels, liver, bones, and joints. Symptoms of late syphilis include slow, progressive loss of muscle coordination, paralysis, blindness, and dementia. If damage to tissues is severe enough, death follows.

Syphilis is diagnosed by a blood test or by laboratory examination of material from the primary chancre or secondary-stage rash. The disease is easily cured with antibiotics, but once damage to internal organs has occurred, there is no way to repair the damage. People who are infected with syphilis are more likely to contract and transmit HIV through sexual contact.

Trichomoniasis and Bacterial Vaginosis

There are many types of **vaginitis**, *an inflammation of the vagina caused by various organisms.* **Trichomoniasis** is *a type of vaginitis caused by the parasite* Trichomonas vaginalis. *It affects both females and males.* Infected males experience symptoms only rarely—irritation inside the penis, mild discharge, or slight burning after urinating or ejaculating. Infected females often have symptoms including a foamy, yellow-green vaginal discharge that has a strong odor. Trichomoniasis in females can also cause genital irritation, itching, and discomfort during intercourse and urination.

Bacterial vaginosis (BV), *a type of vaginitis caused by an imbalance of bacteria normally found in the vagina,* affects only females. Little is known about the cause, but having sexual intercourse with a new partner and douching may be contributing factors.

■ Figure 7.4
The infectious rash of secondary-stage syphilis appears on the palms of the hands and the soles of the feet. *What happens when these external signs disappear?*

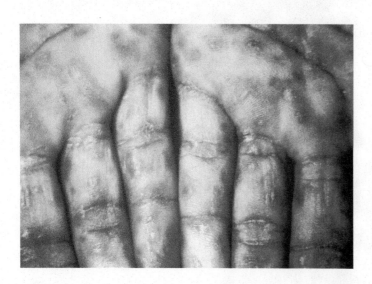

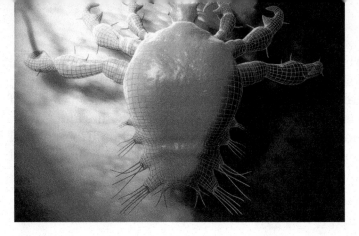

Photo Credit: MedicalRF.com

■ **Figure 7.5**
Special medicated shampoos help eliminate pubic lice.

Symptoms of BV, when present, include white or gray vaginal discharge with a strong odor, as well as itching and burning around the vagina. BV increases the risk of developing gonorrhea and PID, endangering the uterus and fallopian tubes. Both trichomoniasis and BV can make HIV infection more likely.

Pubic Lice

Pubic lice are *tiny parasitic insects, also known as crabs, that infest the genital area of humans.* Pubic lice are usually spread through sexual contact. In rare circumstances, they can spread through infested bed linens, towels, and clothing, since the lice can survive a short time without a host.

The main symptom of lice is intense itching. The lice usually live in pubic hair but can also live in the coarse hair of legs, armpits, mustaches, beards, eyebrows, and eyelashes. Lice that infest the hair on a person's head are not pubic lice.

Special medicated shampoos that kill pubic lice are available over the counter and with a doctor's prescription. These shampoos are harsh and should not be used on the eyebrows or eyelashes. For those areas, a special ointment that will not damage the eyes is available by prescription. Bed linens, towels, and clothing must also be treated to prevent re-infection.

Scabies

Scabies is *an infestation of the skin with microscopic mites called* Sarcoptes scabiei. Scabies is spread by sharing infested bedding and clothing and through prolonged skin-to-skin contact. Scabies is not transmitted by shaking someone's hand.

Symptoms of scabies appear four to six weeks after contact and include a pimple-like rash, particularly between the fingers, in skin folds on the body, and on the penis, breasts, and shoulder blades. The rash causes severe itching, and sores can become infected from scratching.

Did You Know ?

➤ Using a latex condom can provide protection from the spread of certain STDs, including bacterial vaginosis, gonorrhea, chlamydia, syphilis, and HIV. However, it does not protect against all STDs. For example, HSV-2, HPV, pubic lice, and scabies are easily transmitted through contact with an infected area not covered by a condom.

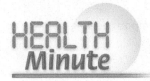

HEALTH Minute

Knowing the Facts Can Help You Make Responsible Decisions

Facts about STDs:

- The body does not build up immunity to STDs, so re-infection can occur.
- Symptoms of some STDs may go away without treatment, but the disease remains in the body.
- It is possible to have an STD without knowing it.

Fewer than ten mites are usually present on an infested person, so diagnosis of scabies can be difficult. Examining the burrows made by the mites provides the best means of diagnosis. All members of infected households, along with all sexual partners of infested people, should be treated at the same time as the infected person by using special lotions that kill the mites.

Treating STDs

STDs can be prevented, and it is every individual's responsibility to practice behaviors that prevent the spread of STDs. Obtaining treatment for STDs is also an important responsibility. STDs will not go away if a person waits long enough; treatment must be sought from a doctor or a public health clinic. For treatment to be successful, a person must do the following:

- Follow the doctor's orders for treatment and take all the medication prescribed. Do not stop taking the medication even if the symptoms have gone away.
- Notify everyone with whom the person has had any sexual contact.
- Remember that abstinence is the only effective method of preventing re-infection or transmission of STDs.

LESSON 2 ASSESSMENT

After You Read
Reviewing Facts and Vocabulary

1. What is *hepatitis B* and how is it transmitted?
2. How is syphilis spread?
3. What occurs in each phase of syphilis?
4. What is the main symptom of pubic lice?
5. What is *scabies*?

Thinking Critically

6. **Synthesize.** Analyze strategies to prevent the spread of syphilis.

7. **Analyze.** Describe the importance and benefits of abstinence. How can teens ensure that they do not contract an STD?

Applying Health Skills

8. **Communication Skills.** Identify, describe, and assess community health services available for the prevention and treatment of STDs. Suppose that a friend came to you and told you that he had a painless sore on the genitals that disappeared within two weeks. What would you advise him to do first? What other advice would you give him?

Reviewing Facts and Vocabulary

1. Which of the following statements is true?

   a. A person can always tell if a sexual partner has an STD.

   b. A person cannot get an STD if he or she has only one sexual partner.

   c. A person could have an STD and not know it.

2. What is the most effective way to avoid getting an STD?

3. Why does chlamydia often go undiagnosed?

4. What is pelvic inflammatory disease? What can result from this STD?

5. How is HPV diagnosed and treated?

6. Why do so many people have HSV-2?

7. Describe the secondary stage of syphilis.

8. How would a doctor determine whether a person has syphilis?

9. Explain how pubic lice are treated.

10. What steps should be taken to treat and prevent the spread of STDs?

Writing Critically

11. **Synthesize.** Write a brief summary describing how STDs are different from most other communicable diseases, such as the common cold, in terms of prevention.

12. **Analyze.** Write a paragraph on whether you think doctors should be required to inform the parents of a patient under the age of 18 who has an STD. Explain your reasons.

13. **Synthesize.** Write a summary describing what might be the consequences if a person infected with an STD never told his sexual partners that he has an STD.

14. **Analyze.** Write a summary explaining why prevention and treatment of STDs is the responsibility of every individual.

Applying Health Skills

15. **Advocacy.** Analyze the importance of abstinence in the prevention of STDs. Write a 30-second radio announcement promoting prevention of STDs in your community.

16. **Analyzing Influences.** Write an essay in which you explain why you think STDs are such a serious problem in the adolescent age group.

Activity Beyond the Classroom

Parent Involvement

Discussing. Discuss with your parents or guardians the issues of STDs, medical information, and privacy for minors under the age of 18. Discuss whether adolescents, adults, or people of any age should be required to inform others if they have an STD.

School and Community

Report to the class. Do research at the library or on the Internet to find further information on a particular STD. Write a report to share with the class. Include symptoms, diagnosis, treatment, and dangers that can occur when the STD is not treated. Include a visual aid when presenting the report to the class.

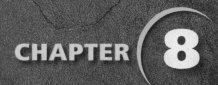

CHAPTER 8

HIV and AIDS

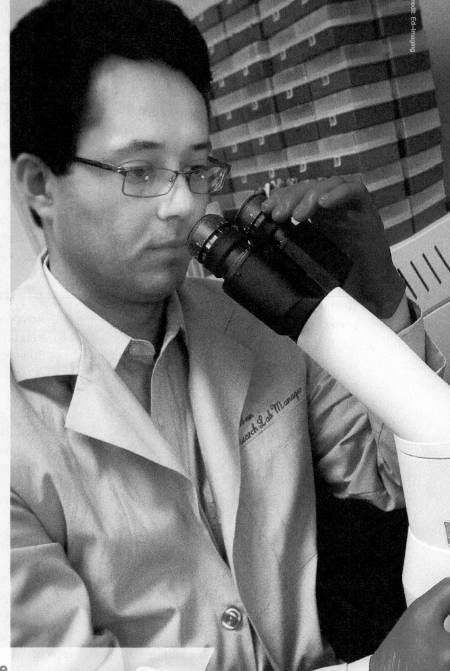

Activating Prior Knowledge

Using Visuals Researchers are working to improve diagnostic methods to identify HIV so that early treatment is possible. List ways you know of in which HIV can be transmitted.

What Is HIV/AIDS?

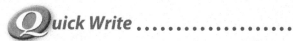

Quick Write ....

> Write a letter to a friend who was sexually active in the past but has been abstinent for more than a year. The friend is now considering being tested for HIV. How would you advise your friend?

Acquired immune deficiency syndrome (AIDS) is *a potentially fatal disorder that interferes with the body's natural ability to fight infection. AIDS is the final stage of infection caused by the **human immunodeficiency virus** (HIV)—a virus that attacks the immune system.*

History and Origin of HIV

The first reported cases of AIDS were diagnosed in the United States in 1981. The earliest identified case of HIV infection dates back to 1959; however, it is possible that the virus may have been infecting humans since 1930 or earlier. Males and females of all races, ages, and sexual orientations can and have become infected with HIV.

How Does HIV Affect the Body?

To understand how HIV attacks the body's immune system, it is necessary to review the functions of lymphocytes. **Lymphocytes** are *specialized white blood cells made in bone marrow that provide the body with immunity*. They help the body fight pathogens, or disease-causing organisms. Two types of lymphocytes protect against diseases: B cells, which mature in bone marrow, and T cells, which mature in the thymus gland. CD4 cells, also called Helper T cells stimulate B cells to produce **antibodies**, which are *proteins that help destroy pathogens that enter the body*.

HIV enters certain cells, including CD4 cells, and reproduces itself. As more cells are infected, more are destroyed. The immune system becomes weakened and is eventually destroyed. The body succumbs to **opportunistic illnesses**, *infections the body could fight off if the immune system were healthy*.

GUIDE TO READING

Building Vocabulary

▸ acquired immune deficiency syndrome (AIDS)
▸ human immunodeficiency virus (HIV)
▸ lymphocytes
▸ antibodies
▸ AIDS-opportunistic illnesses (AIDS-OIs)

Health Concepts

• Identify the stages and symptoms of HIV and AIDS.
• Explain the relationship between risky behaviors and the transmission of HIV.
• Explain why abstinence is the only method that is 100 percent effective in preventing HIV infection.

Reading Strategy

Predict Scan the headings, subheadings, and photo captions. Write down a list of questions you have about HIV/AIDS. After reading the lesson, review your list and fill in the answers.

Photo Credit: ©Kris Timken/Blend Images LLC

HIV can take up to ten years before progressing into AIDS. Researchers are investigating the reasons why a small number of people infected ten or more years ago show no AIDS symptoms. It takes anywhere from three to six weeks after a person is infected to detect the HIV antibodies in their system. This time frame is called the window period. Once detected, HIV usually goes through identifiable stages:

HIV infection moves through identifiable stages before progressing to AIDS:

- **Acute Infection Stage.** This stage begins within two to four weeks of infection. A person may become sick with a severe flu-like illness. Some of the symptoms experienced can include fever, swollen glands, sore throat, rash, muscle and joint aches, fatigue, and headache. During this stage, the virus is reproducing rapidly in the body.

  During the acute infection stage, the levels of HIV in the bloodstream are very high. The virus takes over helper T cells and destroys them. During this stage, the person with HIV can easily transmit the virus to others through sexual activity or drug use, as well as others methods of transmission.

- **Clinical Latency Stage.** During this stage, the HIV virus continues to reproduce in the body, This stage is sometimes referred to as the asymptomatic stage because the person may not feel ill. The clinical latency stage can last for decades if a person is being treated for HIV. For those not being treated, this stage can last for up to an average of 10 years.

- **AIDS.** When the helper T-cells drop to less than 200, or one of several AIDS-opportunistic infections are present, the disease has progressed to the AIDS stage.

■ **Figure 8.1**
All health care workers now wear protective gear to eliminate the risk of contracting or spreading HIV. *Which body fluids are known to carry HIV?*

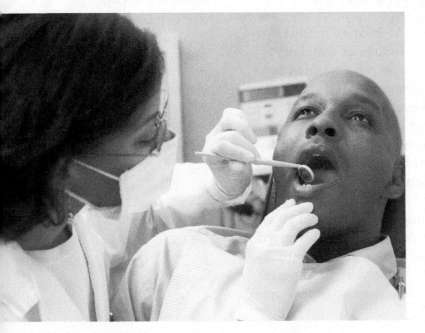

How HIV Is Transmitted

For a person to contract HIV, the virus must enter the individual's blood. HIV is carried in body fluids such as blood, semen, vaginal secretions, and breast milk. A person may come in contact with such infected body fluids and contract the virus if there are breaks in the skin such as cuts, sores, or tiny breaks in the capillaries of mucous membranes. Use of contaminated needles and injected drugs also put a person at risk.

Behaviors Known to Transmit HIV

Certain activities are far more likely than others to transmit HIV. Most of new HIV infections in the United States are contracted in one of two ways: sexual activity with an infected partner and injection drug use:

- **Sexual contact.** Unprotected sexual activity with an infected partner is the main way that HIV is spread. HIV is present in an infected person's vaginal secretions, blood, or semen, and is also present in pre-ejaculatory fluid secreted primarily from the Cowper's glands. During sexual contact, the virus usually enters the body through tiny tears in fragile tissue or breaks in capillaries of mucous membranes. Such tears and breaks are common during genital-genital and anal-genital contact. The larger the number of sex partners a person has, the greater the risk of coming in contact with HIV. People with other STDs that result in sores, bleeding, or discharge are more likely to contract and transmit HIV.

- **Use of contaminated needles.** When a drug user injects drugs with a needle, blood remains on and within the needle after use. If the person is infected with HIV, the virus can be spread to someone else who uses the same needle. Sharing any kind of needles, whether to inject drugs, make tattoos, or do body piercing, puts a person at risk for coming in contact with HIV. Recent studies have found that in addition to needle sharing, people who abuse injection drugs are more likely to engage in high-risk behaviors such as having unprotected sexual intercourse of any kind.

Situations Known to Transmit HIV

If precautions are not followed, HIV can be transmitted whenever blood from an infected person is handled:

- **Blood transfusions.** People who donate blood are not at risk for contracting HIV, because blood donation centers discard needles after each use. Since March 1985, all donated blood in the United States has been tested for HIV. This has almost completely eliminated the risk of contracting HIV from a blood transfusion.

- **Before, during, and after birth.** A pregnant female infected with HIV can pass the virus to her unborn baby through the placenta. During birth, HIV can enter the baby's body through tiny cuts in the skin. After birth, a breast-fed baby can contract HIV from the mother's milk. Approximately one-quarter to one-third of untreated infected females who get pregnant pass the virus on to their babies. Special drugs given to the mother during pregnancy can greatly reduce the baby's risk of contracting HIV. Drug treatment and delivery by cesarean section lowers the risk to about 5 percent.

Did You Know ?

The Ryan White Comprehensive AIDS Resources Emergency (CARE) Act was passed in 1990. It was named for the boy who was infected with HIV at age 13 and died at 18. This act approved funds for AIDS testing, counseling, and treatment for cities and states hardest hit by the disease. Ryan White was one of the first national spokespersons for people with AIDS. Celebrities, musicians, sports personalities, and others continue efforts to raise awareness of the HIV/AIDS issue and advocate for funding and research.

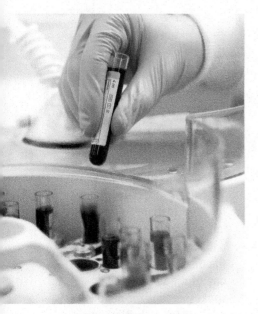

Photo Credit: ©Adam Gault/age fotostock

How HIV Is Not Transmitted

The thought of contracting HIV is frightening, but remember that it can be transmitted only through contact with certain body fluids, including blood, semen, vaginal secretions, and breast milk. HIV cannot be spread through casual contact such as shaking hands, touching, hugging, or kissing. Even within families of an infected individual, HIV is not spread by sharing towels, combs, eating utensils, or bathroom facilities. HIV is not airborne, so it cannot be spread by coughing or sneezing, nor is it transmitted by the bites of insects such as mosquitoes.

■ **Figure 8.2**
Blood that is donated in the United States is tested for HIV.

Teens at Risk

Because sexually active teens tend to engage in high-risk behaviors, they are at serious risk for HIV/AIDS. The CDC gathers statistics on diseases throughout the nation and the world. The following statistics clarify the threat posed by HIV for U.S. teens who engage in high-risk behaviors:

- In 2010, the number of new HIV infections totaled 47,500. Of these, 12,200 or more than 25 percent occurred in people between the ages of 15–29.

- According to the 2011 Youth Risk Behavior Surveillance System report, more than 47 percent of high school students report having had sexual intercourse.

- While condom use among teens who are sexually active has increased, one study shows that 40 percent of high school students report that they did not use a condom the last time they were sexually active.

How can sexually active adults reduce the risk of HIV infection?

Sexually active individuals can take steps to reduce the risk of contracting HIV during sexual intercourse. Having only one partner who is, to the best of their knowledge, not infected with HIV reduces the risk. It is also important to use latex condoms properly during sexual intercourse. Properly used, latex condoms can prevent HIV transmission.

HIV Prevention

Since it was first diagnosed there has been progress in treating AIDS. Many people are living symptom-free for longer periods of time. Today, a mother with HIV has a better chance of not transmitting it to her baby, and people have become educated about the virus and are taking more precautions to protect themselves from coming in contact with it. Despite this progress, HIV/AIDS remains an incurable condition.

Staying Informed

There are many sources of dependable information about HIV infection and AIDS. Reliable sites on the Internet, such as the CDC and other government agencies and medical associations, also offer accurate updates.

During your teen years, you may feel pressure to experiment with new behaviors, such as engaging in sexual activity and/or using alcohol or other drugs. Remember that your decisions will have an impact on the rest of your life, and that the only responsible decision is to choose abstinence from sexual activity, use condoms correctly if you are sexually active, and avoid all drug use, especially injection drug use. Here are some strategies to help you avoid pressure to engage in sexual activity or use drugs:

- Avoid situations in which pressure is almost certain. If you are at a party where the situation is out of control, leave.

- Avoid being alone with a date in a private place. Avoid forming a dating relationship with someone whom you know to be sexually active.

- Avoid the use of alcohol and other drugs. Avoid known drug users and those who approve of drug use.

- When you use refusal strategies, be firm and unwavering. Use body language to reinforce your message.

LESSON 1 ASSESSMENT

After You Read
Reviewing Facts and Vocabulary

1. What is *AIDS* and how is it related to HIV?

2. Describe the asymptomatic stage of AIDS.

3. Explain the relationship between risk behaviors, unsafe situations, and HIV/AIDS. Explain the ways in which HIV is known to be transmitted.

4. Are all teens at serious risk for HIV/AIDS?

Thinking Critically

5. Analyze. Do you think an individual infected with HIV is responsible for informing others of the infection? Why or why not?

6. Synthesize. Why is AIDS a serious threat to public health?

Applying Health Skills

7. Advocacy. Explain why abstinence from alcohol, drugs, and sexual activity is the only method that is 100 percent effective in preventing HIV/AIDS. Design a poster that tells teens how to avoid HIV infection and how to avoid high-risk situations that challenge their decision to abstain from sexual activity and all drug use, especially injection drug use.

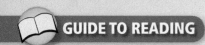
GUIDE TO READING

Building Vocabulary

▶ antibody screening test
▶ Western blot test
▶ pneumocystis carinii pneumonia (PCP)
▶ Kaposi's sarcoma (KS)
▶ cytomegalovirus (CMV)
▶ candidiasis
▶ community outreach programs
▶ grief counselor

Health Concepts

• Describe the tests that are used to diagnose the presence of HIV antibodies.
• Identify the symptoms and medications associated with HIV and AIDS.
• Identify HIV/AIDS support services available in the community.

Reading Strategy

Organize Information Create a graphic organizer showing ways that HIV/AIDS is diagnosed and treated.

HIV/AIDS Testing and Treatment

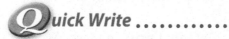

Quick Write ....

Create a two-column chart. In one column, list three or more conditions, careers, or other circumstances that make it important for people to be tested for HIV. Explain your reason for each in the second column.

Within a few years of the diagnosis of the first cases of AIDS in the United States, tests were developed to detect HIV infection. Currently, all donated blood must be tested for HIV. Anyone who donates body organs or tissue, as well as people who join the armed forces, must undergo testing. Medical workers also must undergo testing after occupational exposure to HIV.

Detecting HIV Antibodies

When HIV enters a person's body, the immune system produces antibodies to destroy the pathogen. Unfortunately, the antibodies produced in response to HIV are unable to completely eliminate the virus from the body. HIV tests can detect these antibodies, however, making them useful for diagnosis. It takes an average of 25 days for detectable antibodies to develop, but it may take six months or longer.

Antibody Screening and Confirmatory Tests

The antibody screening test is *a test used to detect the presence of antibodies for HIV in blood*. Results of this tests require three to five days. A more costly test for HIV, called the rapid HIV test, is recommended for use in cases where a person may not return for test results. The rapid test takes about 20 minutes to complete. The rapid test is considered to be highly accurate. However, the results are considered preliminary, and additional tests are needed to confirm the diagnosis.

If the antibody screening test or a rapid HIV test shows a reaction, the test is repeated. If the results are again reactive, a confirmatory test such as the Western blot test is used. The **Western blot test**, is *a specific test that is used in identifying HIV antibodies*. Confirmatory test results generally take one to two weeks. If these results are positive, a person is considered to be infected with HIV. An infected person who may be symptom-free for many years can still infect others when engaging in any activities known to transmit HIV.

Even with a negative result from an antibody screening test or a rapid HIV test, a person might still be infected with HIV because, in some people, it can take the immune system two to four months to develop HIV antibodies. If a person believes she was exposed to HIV and test results are negative, a second test should be performed about six months later. If that test is also negative, the person probably is not infected with HIV. Until the test results are in, however, activities that could transmit the virus must be avoided.

Symptoms of HIV Infection

Many people have no early symptoms when they are infected with HIV, but some develop flu-like symptoms a month or two after they are infected. These symptoms include fever, headache, fatigue, and swollen lymph nodes. Within one to four weeks, these symptoms usually disappear.

A few months to ten years later (or longer), an infected person may develop other symptoms. These include persistent swollen glands, lack of energy, weight loss, frequent fevers and sweats, persistent or frequent yeast infections, skin rashes, and short-term memory loss.

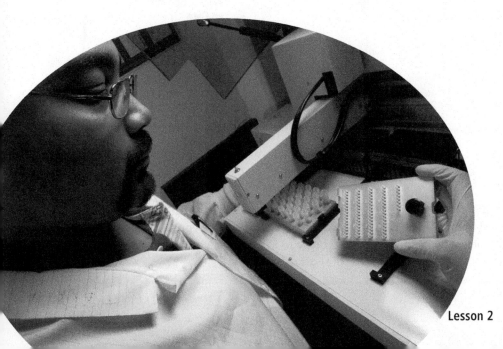

Certain factors can lead to a false-reactive antibody screening test:

- **Laboratory error.** Samples are sometimes incorrectly labeled, or a nonreactive sample is accidentally contaminated by a nearby reactive sample.
- **Blood abnormalities.** Diseases of the blood have been linked to false-reactive tests.
- **Pregnancy.** Women in a second or later pregnancy may have false-reactive readings.
- **Other conditions.** People who have certain conditions such as Lyme disease, syphilis, or lupus may have false-reactive readings.
- **Cross-reactivity with other retroviruses.** Although every virus is different, some viruses have similar genetic makeups. For example, human T cell lymphoma/leukemia viruses (HTLV) have structures similar to that of HIV and therefore produce similar antibodies.

■ **Figure 8.3**
Anyone who has engaged in high-risk behavior should be tested for HIV.

Diagnosis of AIDS

The current CDC definition of AIDS requires that a person be HIV positive *and* have *either* a CD4 cell count below 200 *or* at least one opportunistic illnesses. These are some of the most common opportunistic illnesses.

- **Pneumocystis carinii pneumonia** (PCP), *a fungal infection that causes a form of pneumonia*. This is the most common cause of pneumonia in people with AIDS; symptoms include difficulty breathing, fever, a dry cough, weakness, and weight loss.

- **Kaposi's sarcoma** (KS), *a kind of cancer that develops in connective tissues*. KS usually appears on the skin or in the lining of the mouth, nose, or anus. More serious cases involve the lungs, liver, gastrointestinal tract, and lymph nodes. KS causes flat, painless skin lesions that look like bruises.

Real World CONNECTION

The Cost of HIV/AIDS

The cost of HIV/AIDS in terms of suffering and death is immeasurable. Fortunately, mortality rates in the United States continue to decline. The rate of spending on HIV/AIDS-related issues is not declining, however. Look at the chart below. Which does the government spend more on each year: health care, research, or prevention? Has spending increased more significantly for one area than for another?

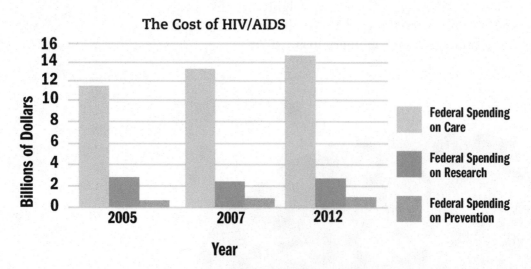

The Cost of HIV/AIDS

Source: CDC. Div. of HIV/AIDS Prevention, Maximizing Impact, DHAP Annual Report 2012.

Activity An estimated 2,369 cases of HIV/AIDS in people in the United States ages 13 through 24 were reported to the CDC in 2005. Research the number of cases reported and the amount of government spending on one other type of STD. Create a graph that compares your findings on the cost of STDs to the cost of HIV/AIDS.

- **Cytomegalovirus** (CMV), *a virus found in 50 percent of the general population and 90 percent of people with HIV.* A weakened immune system allows this opportunistic infection to develop, and it can cause blindness, pneumonia, and gastrointestinal disease.

- **Candidiasis,** *an infection caused by a common type of yeast (fungus) found in almost everyone in the general population.* Genital candidiasis occurs when there is an overgrowth of the fungus *Candida*. Candidiasis can also affect the mouth (thrush) or the throat (esophagitis). Candidiasis of the respiratory tract, trachea, or lungs is related to AIDS.

Research and Treatment

As yet, there is no cure for HIV infection or AIDS. Much progress has been made, however, in delaying the onset of AIDS and in treating opportunistic illnesses.

Drug Research

Antiretroviral drugs inhibit HIV from making copies of itself. The first such drugs developed to fight HIV were zidovudine (AZT), didanosine (ddI), and zalcitabine (ddC). These drugs, known collectively as nucleoside reverse transcriptase inhibitors (NRTIs).

Another class of drugs, called protease inhibitors (PIs), block the progress of HIV in later stages of reproduction within the body. Examples of these drugs are saquinavir, ritonavir, indinavir, and nelfinavir.

Yet a third class of drugs, known as non-nucleoside reverse transcriptase inhibitors (NNRTIs), have also been added to the list of drugs used against AIDS. Examples of these drugs are nevirapine, delavirdine, and efavirenz. Like NRTIs, these drugs keep HIV from infecting new cells. Unfortunately, HIV quickly becomes resistant to NNRTIs when they are used alone.

Scientists discovered that taking a combination of drugs, sometimes referred to as a cocktail, is more effective than taking one drug alone. An assortment of drugs can minimize side effects and prevent HIV from becoming resistant to individual drugs.

Drugs are said to be working if the level of virus in the blood decreases. By using a combination of drugs, some individuals are able to decrease their viral load to such an extent that it is undetectable in blood tests.

What are the major obstacles to research and treatment of HIV/AIDS?

Because HIV is constantly undergoing changes in its genetic structure, the virus has been able to build up resistance to medications. Also, several new strains of HIV have developed, further complicating the search for a vaccine. The treatments that have been developed are very expensive, and some people cannot afford them. In addition, some individuals find it difficult to follow a rigid schedule for taking so many medicines—often with unpleasant side effects— each day.

Vaccines

The search for a vaccine that began in 1987 and a cure for HIV/AIDS continues. Since that time discoveries have led to the development of many drugs that extend the time it takes for HIV to become AIDS. As well as searching for treatments and a cure, the U.S. government has begun a program aimed at reducing the toll of HIV/AIDS.

National HIV/AIDS Strategy

In 2010, the U.S. government introduced the National HIV/AIDS Strategy. The program is aimed at high-risk individuals who know they are HIV-positive, as well as those who are unaware of their status. The program consists of three broad goals:

1. Reduce new HIV infections by providing access to testing and raise awareness of prevention strategies.

2. Increase access to care and improve the health outcomes for people living with HIV. Provide continuous care and permanent housing to all who are HIV-positive.

3. Reduce HIV-related health disparities. This includes increasing access to care.

Support from the Community

People with HIV/AIDS need medical care, but they also need other kinds of support to help them cope with their illness. Extra support often comes from **community outreach programs**, which are *organizations, largely staffed by volunteers, which provide a wide range of essential services to HIV/AIDS patients, their families, and their loved ones.* Community outreach programs provide these services:

- **Practical assistance.** People with HIV/AIDS often need help finding housing as well as getting legal, social, mental health, and visiting-nurse services. Individuals with advanced opportunistic infections may need help making meals.

- **One-on-one support.** Individuals with AIDS may need help with daily activities such as shopping, cooking, and cleaning. Some groups establish a buddy system in which a volunteer helps an individual with daily chores and provides companionship and moral support.

■ **Figure 8.4**
Soup kitchens like this one provide hot meals to people who are homebound with HIV and AIDS.

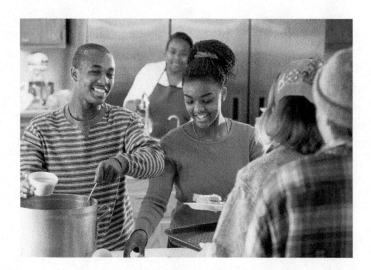

- **Crisis counseling.** Crisis counselors help individuals cope with problems when they feel overwhelmed.
- **Grief counseling.** Most people with HIV/AIDS face a painful, lengthy illness. A **grief counselor** is *a professional who is trained to help people deal with the issues of sickness, dying, and death.* This counselor also can help individuals and their families and loved ones cope with and adjust to the realities of various opportunistic illnesses.
- **Information dissemination.** Those infected with HIV need a way to obtain and interpret the latest accurate information on treatment and care of HIV/AIDS. Many community outreach programs sponsor an AIDS telephone hotline that people can call if they have questions. Some groups, particularly in larger cities, publish newsletters. The San Francisco-based Project Inform sponsors meetings throughout the United States to keep people up to date on the latest information. The CDC keeps a list of community support groups and maintains an AIDS hotline of its own.

LESSON 2 ASSESSMENT

After You Read
Reviewing Facts and Vocabulary

1. What do HIV tests detect?
2. What precautions should a person take if his or her first test results for HIV antibodies are negative?
3. What does the current CDC definition of AIDS require?
4. Identify and describe some of the services provided by community outreach programs for individuals with HIV/AIDS and their families.

Thinking Critically

5. Compare. Explain how technology has impacted the health status of individuals with HIV/AIDS. How are the antibody screening and Western blot tests used?

6. Analyze. Why do you think some people with HIV don't use the recommended combinations of drugs?

Applying Health Skills

7. Advocacy. Prepare a plan for a community outreach program that provides support to people with HIV/AIDS. Provide descriptions of the services that will be provided and information on how teens might get the word out about these services. Include a statement or slogan that would help convince others to join the program and give of their time and talents to help those in need.

Reviewing Facts and Vocabulary

1. How does HIV destroy the immune system?
2. What are *AIDS-opportunistic illnesses*?
3. What is the main way HIV is spread?
4. List three ways HIV is not transmitted.
5. HIV/AIDS is not curable, but it is preventable. What are the best methods of prevention for teens?
6. List possible early symptoms of HIV. How long do they usually last?
7. How long can HIV stay in the body before a person shows symptoms of infection?
8. What is *Kaposi's sarcoma*? What parts of the body are affected in serious cases?
9. How do antiretroviral drugs work?
10. What are *community outreach programs*?

Writing Critically

11. Synthesize. Write an essay explaining why you think many people are uninformed about HIV infection and AIDS.
12. Evaluate. Write a paragraph on whether you believe that people should be required to undergo a test for AIDS before being considered for employment or medical insurance. Explain your reasoning.

13. Analyze. Write a summary analyzing the importance of abstinence from all sexual activity before marriage in reducing the risk of contracting HIV/AIDS. Explain why abstinence from alcohol, drugs, and sexual activity is the only method that is 100 percent effective in preventing HIV/AIDS.
14. Apply. Write a summary explaining the relationship between risk behaviors and HIV/AIDS. A person has been engaging in behaviors that can lead to HIV infection. He has been tested for HIV and the result was negative. What should he do next?

Applying Health Skills

15. Communication Skills. With your parents or guardians, discuss whether you feel HIV testing should be required for health care providers.
16. Refusal Skills. What refusal strategies would you advise a teen to use if her peers were pressuring her to try using an injection drug just one time?

Activity Beyond the Classroom

Parent Involvement
Treating disease. At present, HIV/AIDS is incurable. Many diseases throughout history were also incurable until medical researchers found a way to combat them. With your parent or guardian, choose one of the following diseases and write a report on its history: polio, tuberculosis, pneumonia, bubonic plague, malaria.

School and Community
Local support. Find out what organizations in your community are helping people with AIDS. Make a list of these organizations, and describe specific steps each is taking to help those suffering from AIDS.

— A —

Abortion Any termination of a pregnancy. (Ch. 6, 95)

Abstinence A deliberate decision to avoid harmful behaviors, including sexual activity and the use of alcohol, tobacco, and other drugs. (Ch. 2, 22)

Acquaintance rape Rape by someone the victim knows. (Ch. 6, 98)

Acquired Immune Deficiency Syndrome (AIDS) A potentially fatal disorder that interferes with the body's natural ability to fight infection. AIDS is the final stage of infection caused by the human immunodeficiency virus (HIV). (Ch. 8, 117)

Amniocentesis A procedure that reveals chromosomal abnormalities and certain metabolic disorders in the fetus. (Ch. 5, 75)

Amniotic sac A fluid-filled sac that surrounds the embryo. (Ch. 5, 64)

Antibody screening A test used to detect the presence of antibodies for HIV in blood. (Ch. 8, 122)

Antibodies Proteins that help destroy pathogens that enter the body. (Ch. 8, 117)

— B —

Bacterial vaginosis (BV) A type of vaginitis caused by an imbalance of bacteria normally found in the vagina. (Ch. 7, 112)

Birth defect An abnormality in the structure or function of the body that is present at birth. Birth defects can be caused by abnormal genes or by environmental factors. (Ch. 5, 76)

Birthing centers Facilities that have homelike settings, are separate from a hospital, and offer medication-free births. (Ch. 5, 80)

Bisexual Someone who is sexually attracted to people of both genders. (Ch. 6, 94)

Blastocyst A ball of cells with a cavity in the center. (Ch. 5, 63)

Blended family A family consisting of two married adults who have children from a previous marriage living with them. (Ch. 4, 53)

— C —

Candidiasis An infection caused by a common type of yeast (fungus) found in almost everyone in the general population. (Ch. 8, 125)

Cervical cap A thimble-shaped, soft latex cup that fits snugly over the cervix. (Ch. 6, 86)

Cervix The neck of the uterus. (Ch. 3, 36)

Cesarean birth A method of childbirth in which a surgical incision is made through the abdominal wall and uterus. The baby is lifted out through the surgical incision. (Ch. 5, 78)

Chlamydia An STD that is caused by the bacterium *Chlamydia trachomatis*. (Ch. 7, 106)

Chorionic villi sampling (CVS) A test used to reveal genetic disorders and fetal age and gender. (Ch. 5, 75)

— A —

Aborto Cualquier interrupción de un embarazo.

Abstinencia Una decisión consciente de evitar la conducta peligrosa, como las relaciones sexuales y el uso del alcohol, tabaco y otras drogas.

Violación por un conocido Una violación perpetrada por alguien a quien la víctima conoce.

Síndrome de inmunodeficiencia adquirida (SIDA) Una afección potencialmente mortal que interfiere con la habilidad natural del cuerpo de combatir infecciones. El SIDA es la etapa final de la infección causada por el virus de la inmunodeficiencia humana (VIH).

Amniocentesis Procedimiento que muestra anormalidades en los cromosomas de un feto y ciertos trastornos metabólicos.

Amnios Saco lleno de líquido que rodea el embrión.

Prueba de detección de anticuerpos Prueba para detectar la presencia de anticuerpos contra el VIH en la sangre.

Anticuerpos Proteínas que ayudan a destruir los patógenos gérmenes que entran en el cuerpo.

— B —

Vaginosis bacteriana Un tipo de vaginosis causada por el desequilibrio de bacterias que normalmente están en la vagina.

Defecto de nacimiento Anormalidad en la estructura o función del cuerpo que está presente al nacimiento. Puede ser el resulto de genes anormales o de factores ambientales.

Centros de parto natural Instalaciones que tienen un ambiente hogareño, están separados de los hospitales y ofrecen partos sin medicación.

Bisexual Alguien que siente atracción sexual por personas de ambos géneros.

Blastocisto Un balón de células con una cavidad en el centro.

Familia mixta Una familia en que se casan dos adultos que tienen hijos de un matrimonio anterior viviendo con ellos.

— C —

Candidiasis Infección por un tipo común de levadura (hongos) que está presente en casi toda la gente.

Tapón cervical Una tapa de látex blanda en forma de dedal que se calza por encima de la apertura del útero o cérvix.

Cerviz Cuello del útero.

Parto por cesárea Un método de parto en el que se hace una incisión quirúrgica a través de la pared abdominal y el útero. El bebé se saca a través de la incisión.

Clamidia Una enfermedad de transmisión sexual causada por la bacteria *Chlamydia trachomatis*.

Biopsia de vellosidades coriónicas Prueba utilizada para mostrar trastornos genéticos y la edad y el género del feto.

Cognitive Relating to the ability to reason and think out abstract solutions. (Ch. 1, 8)

Commitment A promise or a pledge. (Ch. 4, 49)

Communication The process through which you send messages to and receive messages from others. (Ch. 2, 19)

Community outreach programs Organizations, largely staffed by volunteers, which provide a wide range of essential services to HIV/AIDS patients, their families, and their loved ones. (Ch. 8, 126)

Condom A thin sheath of latex, plastic, or animal tissue that is placed on the erect penis to catch semen. It is a physical barrier to the passage of sperm into the vagina and toward the ovum. (Ch. 6, 85)

Conflict A disagreement, struggle, or fight. (Ch. 2, 20)

Contraception Prevention of pregnancy. (Ch. 6, 84)

Contraceptive injection A birth control procedure in which a female receives an injection once every three months to prevent ovulation. (Ch. 6, 89)

Cytomegalovirus (CMV) A virus found in 50 percent of the general population and 90 percent of people with HIV. (Ch. 8, 125)

———————————— **D** ————————————

Date rape Rape by someone the victim is dating. (Ch. 6, 98)

Developmental tasks An event that needs to occur during a particular age period for a person to continue his or her growth toward becoming a healthy, mature adult. (Ch. 1, 8)

Diaphragm A soft latex or silicone cup with a flexible rim that covers the entrance to the cervix. (Ch. 6, 86)

———————————— **E** ————————————

Embryo An implanted blastocyst from the time of implantation until about the eighth week of development. (Ch. 5, 64)

Empathy The ability to feel what others feel, to put yourself in someone else's place. (Ch. 1, 11)

Endocrine system A body system made up of ductless glands that secrete chemicals called hormones into the blood. (Ch. 1, 12)

Epididymis A highly coiled structure located on the back side of each testis. (Ch. 3, 30)

Episiotomy An incision made from the vagina toward the anus to enlarge the opening for delivery of a baby. (Ch. 5, 77)

———————————— **F** ————————————

Fallopian tubes Tubes on each side of the uterus that connect the uterus to the region of the ovaries. (Ch. 3, 37)

Fertility awareness methods (FAMs) Methods of contraception that involve determining the fertile days of the female's menstrual cycle and avoiding intercourse during those days. (Ch. 6, 84)

Fertilization The union of a single sperm and an ovum.(Ch. 5, 63)

Fetal alcohol syndrome (FAS) A condition of physical, mental, and behavioral abnormalities that can result when a pregnant female drinks alcohol. (Ch. 5, 73)

Fetus A developing baby from the end of the eighth week after fertilization until birth. (Ch. 5, 65)

Cognitivo Referente a la capacidad para pensar y llegar a soluciones abstractas.

Compromiso Un acuerdo o promesa.

Comunicación Proceso por el cual envías mensajes y recibes mensajes de otros.

Programas para ayudar a la comunidad Organizaciones dirigidas mayormente por voluntarios quienes proveen servicios esenciales para las personas con VIH/SIDA, sus familias y otros seres queridos.

Condón Una lámina fina de plástico, látex o tejido animal que se coloca en el pene erecto para recoger semen. Actúa como una barrera física, impidiendo que el semen entre en la vagina o pase hacia el óvulo.

Conflicto Desacuerdo, lucha o pelea.

Anticoncepción La prevención de embarazos.

Inyección anticonceptivo Un proceso anticonceptivo en el cual una mujer recibe una inyección una vez cada tres meses para prevenir la ovulación.

Citomegalovirus (CMV) Virus que se encuentra en 50 por ciento del gran público y en 90 por ciento de la gente con VIH.

———————————— **D** ————————————

Violación durante una cita (violación a escondidas) Violación por alguien con quien la víctima sale.

Tareas requeridas para el desarrollo Un suceso que tiene que ocurrir a una edad determinada para que la persona pueda continuar su desarrollo hasta la madurez saludable.

Diafragma Un disco de látex o silicio blando con borde flexible que cubre la apertura del útero.

———————————— **E** ————————————

Embrión Un blastocisto implantado, desde el momento de implantación hasta aproximadamente la octava semana de desarrollo.

Empatía La capacidad de sentir lo que otros sienten, de ponerse en el lugar de otro.

Sistema endocrino Un sistema del cuerpo compuesto de glándulas sin conductos que secretan sustancias químicas llamadas hormonas en la sangre.

Epidídimo Una estructura en forma de madeja u ovillo ubicada detrás de cada testículo.

Episiotomía Una incisión hecha desde la vagina hacia el ano para agrandar el orificio vaginal durante el parto de un bebé.

———————————— **F** ————————————

Trompas de Falopio Los tubos a ambos lados del útero que conectan el útero a la región de los ovarios.

Métodos anticonceptivos de abstinencia en días fértiles Métodos anticonceptivos que implican la determinación de los días fértiles en el ciclo menstrual de la mujer para no tener relaciones sexuales durante esos días.

Fertilización La unión de un espermatozoide con un óvulo.

Síndrome de alcoholismo fetal (SAF) Anormalidades físicas, mentales y de comportamiento que pueden ocurrir cuando una mujer embarazada toma alcohol.

Feto Un bebé en desarrollo, desde el fin de la octava semana después de fertilización hasta el nacimiento.

G

Genes Units of heredity that determine which traits, or characteristics, offspring inherit from their parents. (Ch. 5, 67)

Genetic counseling A process in which the genetic histories of prospective parents are studied to determine the presence of certain hereditary diseases. (Ch. 5, 68)

Genital herpes An STD caused by the herpes simplex virus. Herpes simplex 1 usually causes cold sores in or near the mouth. (Ch. 7, 107)

Genital warts Soft, moist, pink or red swellings that appear on the genitals and are caused by the human papillomavirus. (Ch. 7, 105)

Goal Something you aim for that takes planning and work. (Ch. 1, 7)

Gonorrhea An STD caused by bacteria that live in warm, moist areas of the body, such as mucous membranes. (Ch. 7, 106)

Grief counselor A professional who is trained to help people deal with the issues of sickness, dying, and death. (Ch. 8, 127)

H

Hepatitis B (HBV) A viral STD that attacks the liver and can cause extreme illness and death. (Ch. 7, 110)

Heredity Genetic characteristics passed from parent to child. (Ch. 4, 55)

Heterosexual Someone who is sexually attracted to people of the opposite gender. (Ch. 6, 94)

Homosexual Someone who is sexually attracted to people of the same gender. (Ch. 6, 94)

Hormones Chemical substances produced in glands, which regulate the activities of different body cells and organs. (Ch. 1, 12; Ch. 3, 44)

Human immunodeficiency virus (HIV) A virus that attacks the immune system. (Ch. 8, 117)

Human papillomavirus (HPV) A virus that causes genital warts and warts on other parts of the body. (Ch. 7, 105)

I

Incest Sexual contact between family members who cannot marry by law. (Ch. 6, 96)

Intersexual An individual who was born with both male and female characteristics. (Ch. 6, 94)

Intimacy A closeness between two people that develops over time. (Ch. 2, 24)

K

Kaposi's sarcoma (KS) A kind of cancer that develops in connective tissues. (Ch. 8, 124)

L

Labor The process by which contractions gradually push the baby out of the uterus and into the vagina to be born. (Ch. 5, 77)

LGBTQ Lesbian, gay, bisexual, transgender, or questioning. (Ch. 6, 94)

Lymphocytes Specialized white blood cells made in bone marrow that provide the body with immunity. (Ch. 8, 117)

G

Genes Unidades de herencia que determinan qué rasgos o características los hijos heredan de los padres.

Asesoría genética Proceso en el que se estudian las historias genéticas de los que quieren ser padres para determinar la presencia de ciertas enfermedades hereditarias.

Herpes genital Enfermedad de transmisión sexual causada por el virus del herpes simple. Normalmente, el herpes simple 1 produce llagas frías en la boca o cerca de esta.

Verrugas genitales Hinchazones blandas, rosadas o rojas e húmedas que aparecen en los órganos genitales. Son el resultado del virus del papiloma humano.

Meta Algo que quieres alcanzar que requiere planificación y trabajo.

Gonorrea Una enfermedad de transmisión sexual causada por bacterias que viven en las zonas cálidas y húmedas del cuerpo, por ejemplo las membranas mucosas.

Consejero del duelo Profesional que ayuda a la gente con los asuntos de la enfermedad y la muerte.

H

Hepatitis B Enfermedad viral de transmisión sexual que ataca el hígado y puede causar otras enfermedades graves o la muerte.

Herencia Características genéticas transmitidas de padres a hijos.

Heterosexual Alguien que siente atracción sexual por personas del sexo opuesto.

Homosexual Alguien que siente atracción sexual por personas del mismo sexo.

Hormonas Sustancias químicas que se producen en las glándulas y regulan la actividad de distintas células y órganos del cuerpo.

Virus de la inmunodeficiencia humana (VIH) Un virus que ataca el sistema inmune.

Virus del papiloma humano (VPH) Virus que causa verrugas genitales y verrugas en otras partes del cuerpo.

I

Incesto Contacto sexual entre miembros de una familia que no pueden casarse por ley.

Intersexual Una persona que nació con características tanto masculinas como femeninas.

Intimidad Un sentimiento de cercanía entre dos personas que se desarrolla a lo largo del tiempo.

K

Sarcoma de Kaposi (SK) Tipo de cáncer que se desarrolla en el tejido conectivo.

L

Trabajo de parto El proceso por el cual contracciones gradualmente empujan el bebé fuera del útero hacia la vagina para nacer.

LGBTQ Lesbiana, gay, bisexual, trangénero, o cuestionamiento

Linfocitos Glóbulos blancos especializados que se producen en la médula ósea y proporcionan inmunidades al cuerpo.

M

Masturbation Touching one's own genitals for sexual pleasure. (Ch. 6, 93)

Menstruation The process of shedding the uterine lining. (Ch. 3, 38)

O

Opportunistic illnesses Infections the body could fight off if the immune system were healthy. (Ch. 8, 118)

Oral contraceptives Hormone pills that, taken correctly, create changes in the female body that prevent pregnancy. (Ch. 6, 88)

Ovaries The two female sex glands, which produce mature ova and female hormones. (Ch. 3, 37)

Ovulation The process of releasing one mature ovum each month into a fallopian tube. (Ch. 3, 37)

P

Parenting Providing care, support, and love in a way that leads to a child's total development. (Ch. 4, 56)

Peer pressure The influence that people your own age may have on you. (Ch. 2, 18)

Pelvic inflammatory disease (PID) A painful infection of the uterus, fallopian tubes, and/or ovaries. (Ch. 7, 106)

Penis A tubelike organ that functions in both sexual reproduction and the elimination of urine. (Ch. 3, 30)

Pituitary gland The gland that controls much of the endocrine system. It releases hormones that affect the brain, glands, skin, bones, muscles, and reproductive organs. (Ch. 1, 13)

Placenta A structure that forms along the lining of the uterus as the embryo implants. (Ch. 5, 64)

Pneumocystis carinii pneumonia (PCP) A fungal infection that causes a form of pneumonia. (Ch. 8, 124)

Prenatal Occurring or existing before birth. (Ch. 5, 69)

Puberty The period of growth from physical childhood to physical adulthood, when a person develops certain traits of his or her own gender. (Ch. 1, 12)

Pubic lice Tiny parasitic insects, also known as crabs, that infest the genital area of humans. (Ch. 7, 113)

R

Rape Any form of sexual intercourse that takes place against a person's will. (Ch. 6, 98)

Refusal skills Communication strategies that help you say no effectively when you are urged to take part in behaviors that are unsafe or unhealthful, or go against your values. (Ch. 2, 26)

Rubella (German measles) A contagious disease caused by a virus that does not cause serious complications except in pregnancy. (Ch. 5, 73)

S

Scabies An infestation of the skin with microscopic mites called *Sarcoptes scabiei*. (Ch. 7, 113)

Scrotum A loose sac of skin that extends outside the body and contains the testes. (Ch. 3, 29)

M

Masturbación Tocarse los propios órganos genitales para obtener placer sexual.

Menstruación El proceso de desprendimiento del revestimiento del útero.

O

Enfermedades oportunistas Infecciones que el cuerpo podría combatir si el sistema inmune estuviera sano.

Anticonceptivos orales Pastillas de hormonas que, cuando se toman correctamente, hacen cambios en el cuerpo de una mujer que impiden el embarazo.

Ovarios Las dos glándulas sexuales femeninas que producen óvulos maduros y las hormonas sexuales femeninas.

Ovulación La liberación de un óvulo maduro cada mes en una trompa de Falopio.

P

Crianza Proveer cuidado, apoyo y amor de tal manera que conduzca al desarrollo total de un niño.

Presión de los compañeros La influencia que tus contemporáneos pueden tener sobre ti.

Enfermedad inflamatoria pélvica (EIP) Una infección dolorosa del útero, de las trompas de Falopio y/o de los ovarios.

Pene Un órgano tubular que funciona en la reproducción sexual y la eliminación de la orina.

Glándula pituitaria La glándula que controla gran parte del sistema endocrino. Secreta otras hormonas que afectan el cerebro, otras glándulas, la piel, los huesos, los músculos y los órganos reproductores.

Placenta Una estructura que se forma a lo largo del revestimiento del útero al implantarse el embrión.

Neumonía por pneumocystis carinii (NPC) Una infección de hongos que causa un forma de neumonía.

Prenatal Que ocurre o existe antes del nacimiento.

Pubertad El período de crecimiento entre la infancia y la edad adulta desde el punto de vista físico cuando una persona desarrolla ciertas características de su propio género.

Ladillas Pequeñitos insectos parasíticos que infestan el vello púbico de personas.

R

Violación Cualquier tipo de relación sexual que ocurre contra la voluntad de la persona.

Habilidades de negación Estrategias de comunicación que te ayudan a decir que no cuando alguien te anima a participar en conducta que no es sana, es peligrosa, o está en contra de tus valores.

Rubéola (sarampión Alemana) Enfermedad contagiosa causada por un virus que no tiene gran trascendencia, menos durante el embarazo.

S

Sarna Afección de la piel causada por insectos aradores muy pequeños que se llaman *Sarcoptes scabiei*.

Escroto Un saco suelto de piel externo al cuerpo que contiene los testículos.

Self-concept The mental image you have about yourself. It is your unique set of perceptions, ideas, and attitudes about yourself. (Ch. 1, 5)

Semen A mixture of sperm and glandular secretions. (Ch. 3, 30)

Sexual abuse Any sexual contact that is physically or emotionally forced on a person against his or her will. (Ch. 6, 96)

Sexuality Everything about you as a male or female. It includes the way you act, your personality, and how you feel about yourself because you are male or female. (Ch. 1, 4)

Sexually transmitted diseases (STDs) Infections that spread from person to person through sexual contact. (Ch. 7, 103)

Single-parent family A family that consists of only one parent and one or more children. (Ch. 4, 58)

Sperm The male reproductive cells. (Ch. 3, 29)

Spermicide A chemical that kills sperm. (Ch. 6, 85)

Stereotype An idea or image held about a group of people that represents a prejudiced attitude, oversimplified opinion, or uninformed judgment. (Ch. 6, 94)

Syphilis An STD caused by the bacterium *Treponema pallidum;* it progresses in stages. (Ch. 7, 111)

— **T** —

Testes The male sex glands, which produce sperm and manufacture testosterone. (Ch. 3, 29)

Testosterone The male sex hormone produced by the testes. (Ch. 3, 29)

Transgender An individual whose gender identity differs from others of their gender. (Ch. 6, 93)

Trichomoniasis A type of vaginitis caused by the parasite *Trichomonas vaginalis.* It affects both females and males. (Ch. 7, 112)

Tubal ligation A sterilization procedure for females in which the fallopian tubes are cut and tied or clamped to prevent sperm from reaching the ova. (Ch. 6, 92)

— **U** —

Ultrasound A test that produces an image on a screen by reflecting sound waves off the body's inner structures. (Ch. 5, 75)

Umbilical cord A ropelike structure that connects the embryo and the mother's placenta. (Ch. 5, 64)

Uterus A hollow, muscular organ that receives, holds, and nourishes the fertilized ovum during pregnancy. (Ch. 3, 36)

— **V** —

Vagina An elastic, muscle-lined tube that extends from the uterus to outside the body and is also called the birth canal. (Ch. 3, 36)

Vaginitis An inflammation of the vagina caused by various organisms. (Ch. 7, 112)

Values The beliefs and standards of conduct that are important to a person. (Ch. 2, 17)

Vas deferens A long tube that connects each epididymis with the urethra. (Ch. 3, 31)

Auto-concepto La imagen mental que tienes de ti mismo. Es tu conjunto único de percepciones, ideas y actitudes sobre ti mismo.

Semen La mezcla de esperma y fluidos de las glándulas.

Abuso sexual Cualquier contacto sexual, física o emocionalmente, forzado contra la voluntad de una persona.

Sexualidad Todo lo que se refiere a ti como hombre o mujer. Incluye la forma en que actúas, tu personalidad y tus sentimientos respecto de ti mismo por ser hombre o mujer.

Enfermedades de transmisión sexual (ETS) Infecciones que se transmiten de persona en persona a través del contacto sexual.

Familias de un solo padre Una familia compuesta por un sólo padre y uno o más niños.

Esperma Las células reproductoras masculinas.

Espermicida Un producto químico que mata a las espermas.

Estereotipo Una idea o imagen acerca de un grupo de personas que representa una actitud prejuiciosa, una opinión simplista o un juicio sin fundamento.

Sífilis Enfermedad de transmisión sexual causada por la bacteria llamada *Treponema pallidum.* La enfermedad progresa en etapas.

— **T** —

Testículos Las glándulas sexuales masculinas que producen esperma y testosterona.

Testosterona La hormona sexual masculina producida por los testículos.

Transgénero Un individuo cuya identidad de género difiere de otros de su género

Tricomoniasis Un tipo de vaginitis causada por el parásito llamado Trichomonas *vaginalis.* Afecta a mujeres y a hombres.

Ligadura de trompas Procedimiento de esterilización para mujeres en que las trompas de Falopio se cortan y se atan o cierran para impedir que el espermatozoide llegue a los óvulos.

— **U** —

Ultrasonido (ecografía) Un examen que produce una imagen en una pantalla al reflejar las ondas de sonido que chocan contra las estructuras internas del cuerpo.

Cordón umbilical Una estructura como una cuerda que conecta el embrión con la placenta de la madre.

Útero Un órgano hueco y muy musculoso que recibe, mantiene y nutre el óvulo fecundado durante el embarazo.

— **V** —

Vagina Una vía tubular, elástica y muscular que se extiende desde el útero hasta afuera del cuerpo. También se llama el canal de parto.

Vaginitis Una inflamación de la vagina causada por varios organismos.

Valores Creencias y normas de conducta que son importantes para una persona.

Conductos deferentes Un tubo largo que conecta el epidídimo con la uretra.

Vasectomy A sterilization procedure for males in which each vas deferens is cut and sealed. (Ch. 6, 91)

Vulva External female reproductive organs. They consist of the mons pubis, labia majora (outer lips), labia minora (inner lips), vaginal opening, and clitoris. (Ch. 3, 35)

W

Western blot test A specific test that is used in identifying HIV antibodies. (Ch. 8, 123)

Withdrawal The male's removal of the penis from the vagina before ejaculation. (Ch. 6, 84)

Z

Zygote A fertilized ovum. (Ch. 5, 63)

Vasectomía Un procedimiento de esterilización para hombres en que los conductos deferentes se cortan y se cierran.

Vulva Los órganos externos del sistema reproductor femenino. Consisten en el monte de Venus, los labios mayores y los labios menores, el orificio vaginal y el clítoris.

W

Western blot test Prueba muy específica para identificar los anticuerpos contra el VIH.

Coito interrupto La extracción del pene por el hombre de la vagina antes de la eyaculación.

Z

Cigoto (zigoto) Un óvulo fertilizado.